When
Your Baby
Won't Stop
Crying

When Your Baby Won't Stop Crying

A Parent's Guide to Colic

Tonja H. Krautter
Psy.D., L.C.S.W.

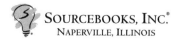

SOURCEBOOKS, INC.®
NAPERVILLE, ILLINOIS

Published by Sourcebooks, Inc.
P.O. Box 4410, Naperville, Illinois 60567-4410
(630) 961-3900
Fax: (630) 961-2168
www.sourcebooks.com

Library of Congress Cataloging-in-Publication Data

Krautter, Tonja H.
    When your baby won't stop crying : a parent's guide to colic / Tonja H. Krautter.
        p. cm.
    ISBN-13: 978-1-4022-0675-7
    ISBN-10: 1-4022-0675-5
    1. Colic. 2. Crying in infants. 3. Infants (Newborn)—Care. I. Title.
    RJ267.K73 2006
    618.92'09755—dc22
                                                    2005037936

Printed and bound in the United States of America
VP 10 9 8 7 6 5 4 3 2 1

I dedicate this book to my beautiful baby boy,
Tyler Krautter Pearson.
Our journey together has created a bond
between us that cannot be broken.
You are my light; you are my miracle.

I have written this book in hopes that our story
will help individuals who have difficult infants
endure their struggles with less stress and anxiety
and more understanding from those around them.

Contents

Foreword

Perhaps you are one of the worried parents who has just had a baby who is everything you hoped for—except he is colicky. He looks just perfect, but something seems to be very wrong. You consult everyone you know, desperate for help and advice. Your pediatrician assures you there is nothing really wrong with the baby. You do your best to comfort your child, but he remains inconsolable. No matter what you do, your baby won't stop crying.

Under the best of circumstances, rearing a child is challenging. As the parent of a colicky baby, you face additional challenges that seem overwhelming. You are sleep-deprived and confused. You feel helpless and perhaps even hopeless. You doubt yourself and wonder what's wrong with *you*.

It can happen to anyone. Although heredity seems to play a part, in most cases the cause of this unexpected challenge cannot be pinpointed. Any parent can be confronted with a child with colic. Whatever your parenting situation, whatever your background, whether your circumstances are ideal or devastating, it does not matter to a child with colic.

Thankfully, you are not alone. Dr. Tonja Krautter, a clinical psychologist with years of experience in child, adolescent, and family therapy, has also gone through the devastating experience of raising a baby with colic. In her quest for solutions, she discovered that no parenting books address this problem adequately. She found that among the few clinical solutions that address the problem, none are sure to help address the physical and emotional impact on the parents and the family. *When Your Baby Won't Stop Crying: A Parent's Guide to Colic* will help you and yours to recognize, understand, and find some practical solutions to calm the colicky infant.

When Your Baby Won't Stop Crying: A Parent's Guide to Colic is both easy to read and packed with strategies and concrete tools that will apply to all fussy babies. Dr. Krautter also speaks to the emotional pain parents go through as they attempt to console their newborn child. This comprehensive, well-researched volume offers detailed advice. The reader will notice specific guidance when they need it and will be touched personally. Rather than go through the ordeal alone, here is the sound advice you need from a mental health professional who has been in your shoes.

—Rebecca A. Powers, MD

Acknowledgments

I am a practicing clinical psychologist who finds great meaning in helping others. I feel honored and privileged to work in the mental health field. In addition, I am a mother who finds great meaning in raising two precious children. Both my family and my career are priorities in my life. I feel blessed to have created a balance between them.

Colic is a highly misunderstood phenomenon, which can leave a family feeling frustrated, confused, and defeated. My greatest hope in writing this book is to provide validation to all the families who are currently struggling with a colicky infant and those who have struggled with one in the past.

I would like to acknowledge the contributions of several people, without whom I would not have completed this book.

To my colleagues who provided me with suggestions and feedback on my written material while in the developmental stages of the book: Fawn Powers, James Lock, Rebecca Powers, and Anthony Atwell.

To my good friend, Phil Schaaf, who through his guidance, support, and inspiration was fundamental in getting this project off the ground.

To my agent, Jodie Rhodes, for believing in my story and having the vision to help me share it with others. To Sourcebooks for their interest in my story. To my editor, Deb Werksman, for her hard work and commitment to the final product. To Rachel Jay for her help with the final touches.

To the many people who supported me in my efforts and convinced me that this book was a must-read for other families who have walked in my family's shoes: Gale and John Uhl, Andrea and Scott Ancha, Nicole and Anthony Radalj, Chris Memoli, Katy and Devin Samaha, Alison and Dean Cappelazzo, Janice and Steve O'Deagan, Kathy Likens, Susan Schick, Valerie Mulhollen, Pamela Rennert, Morton Berman, Karen Parrish, Laura and Don Stemmle, Pat Bonasera, Narisse Kendrick, and all my colleagues in private practice.

To my mother, Heidi Krautter, who stood by me during the toughest months of Tyler's colic without complaint and with unconditional support. To my father, Alfred Krautter, who motivated me to persevere not only during the colicky months, but thereafter in my book-writing ventures. To my grandmother, Hermine Krautter, who taught me that with hard work, perseverance, and commitment you can accomplish anything. To my brother, Torsten Krautter, who reminded me that humor can help in the toughest of times. To my in-laws, Nanette and Roger Pearson, who kept reminding me that things *would* get better. To my brother-in-law, Josh Pearson, and my aunt, Norma Weisbrich, who consistently validated our struggles. To my brother-in-law, Ryan Pearson, and my sister-in-law, Sara Pearson, who offered kind words, support, and encouragement.

To my incredible husband and soul mate, Jason Rockwell Pearson, whose constant encouragement and reassurance during the development of this book was invaluable. His unconditional love and support throughout our journey of raising a colicky baby both inspired me to write this book and to help others who have walked in our shoes.

Thank you all!

Introduction

Prior to having my first child, a friend told me, "Parenthood is like a roller coaster. You know that there are ups and downs...you just don't always see them coming." After eighteen months of raising a child with an extreme case of colic, I reminded her of our conversation and amended her assessment. "Parenthood is like a roller coaster," I agreed, "but parenting a colicky infant is like a roller coaster that can derail at any time."

What You Will Learn from This Book

The purpose of this book is to help you better understand how to assess, diagnose, and treat colic. It details the psychological ramifications that present themselves when your baby simply won't stop crying. Unfortunately, colic is a highly complex and confusing problem that affects both the baby and his or her family. The colicky baby is hard to soothe at best and the colicky infant's parents are distraught over the infant's relentless cries. It is not uncommon for parents to feel helpless as caregivers and hopeless in finding a solution. Therefore, the solutions provided are to help both the baby and the parent decrease their ongoing distress.

Parenthood is not easy. Most first-time parents are simultaneously consumed with feelings of both excitement and fear. Not knowing what to expect can rattle even the most solid individual. People say to "expect the unexpected," but it is impossible to absorb the context of this old adage. As a clinical psychologist who has worked for years on extreme-case matters involving abuse, violence, and suicide, I like to think that I am prepared for the unexpected. Or rather, that the unexpected does not surprise me. Having an infant with colic quickly challenged these beliefs.

I was inspired to write this book for three main reasons. Colic is still largely a misunderstood condition, yet one that impacts millions of families. According to several sources (i.e., colichelp.com and thenewparentsguide.com), an estimated one million babies are born each year with some form of colic. Given that approximately four million children are born each year, 25 percent of American families are currently impacted by some form of the condition.

The first formal medical definition of colic was developed by Dr. Morris Wessel, a pediatrician based in Connecticut. He defined colic as the "Rule of Threes." In short, if an infant cries at least three hours a day, three days per week, for three weeks in a row, then he or she is considered to be suffering from colic. Colic usually starts when the baby is two weeks old and ends when the baby is one hundred days old. However, some infants start to struggle with this problem earlier and experience it for a longer period of time. For example, my son's inconsolable crying began in the hospital soon after he was born and lasted for six months.

Although there is no known cure for colic, it can be improved with soothing techniques such as offering the baby something to suck on, singing, holding, rocking, white noise, and massage. These strategies and many more will be described in greater detail in later chapters. I find it important to note that even though these interventions are clearly more old wives' tales than scientific truisms, thousands of families all over the world utilize them successfully to soothe their crying baby.

The more scientific approaches to the problem of colic are also described in later chapters. These theories focus on the physiology of the body: specifically the stomach and the brain. For example, one scientific theory identifies two different types of stomach problems that are presumed to be the main culprit in colic; the immature baby's digestive system and abdominal pain due to intestinal illness, such as stomach acid reflux or food intolerance/allergy. The other scientific theory identifies what is considered to be the "underdeveloped infant brain," which causes the baby to cry uncontrollably due to overstimulation in his environment.

Two more theories of colic are investigated in later chapters. One is based on parental anxiety and the other is based on the baby's temperament. Both are proposed to be the root cause of colic and a primary factor in the maintenance of this problem. All of the theories listed above are explored and challenged on their reliability, validity, and conclusiveness.

The second source of inspiration to write this book stemmed from something I learned in my profession: overly stressed individuals need a means to relieve the tension that builds within them. And this certainly applies to parents with problematic infants. The combination of high-stress conditions, sleep deprivation, and frustration can lead to a cycle of negativity that has destructive consequences for everyone in the family unit. Furthermore, the intense feelings of hopelessness and helplessness can catalyze impulsive behaviors which, in a more rational state of mind, parents would never consider.

In 2002, 896,000 children were determined to be victims of child abuse or neglect. There were 1,400 infant fatalities due to abuse or neglect in 2003. That is 1.98 children per 100,000 children in our country. Children under one year of age accounted for 41 percent of these fatalities. Did these parents have difficult children and few or no resources with which to cope? Even if the answer is yes, certainly this does not excuse their behavior. However, this information can give us some insight into why it occurred, and that information can potentially help us prevent similar situations from occurring in the future with people who are in similar circumstances.

I am not suggesting that colic is the root cause for abuse, neglect, and infanticide, but it can present an unnerving challenge resulting in a parent's impaired judgment. As someone who recommends coping mechanisms to hundreds of adults every year, I found it revealing to see myself in an unhinged environment grasping for the proverbial rope. Admittedly, there were times I felt comprehensively defeated, but I was saved by my professional and personal belief in problem solving.

Mental health professionals constantly search for creative ways to help reduce their patients' isolation and help them to gain the support necessary to feel better understood. Suffice it to say, hearing from others' experiences with colicky infants could diminish the devastation that the parents and their family members face on a day-to-day basis. Furthermore, gaining knowledge of how parents with colicky infants cope with the immense stress they are under could decrease the potential for abuse and infant death. Perhaps with this recognition, parents with few resources could obtain the necessary tools to prevent isolation, despair, and trauma.

The third and most important reason for writing this book is to offer some tangible explanations and relief to those confronted by colic. I offer a psychological perspective on infant crying and discuss how individuals can cope with distress. I also discuss the consequences of sleep deprivation and review the clinical signs and symptoms of postpartum depression with a list of strategies that I utilized to combat the postpartum "blues." Resources for readers who are currently struggling with postpartum depression are also listed.

In addition, I detail the many attempts my family made to stop my baby's crying. These strategies and interventions are presented in order to give the reader some initial options and ideas to resolve problematic crying and hopefully help the newborn to sleep longer. I know that there are millions of people who have traveled the same path as my family, and millions more to come. I hope that the struggles of our journey through the mystifying and relentless world of colic might somehow offer hope and solace to them.

My Story

Like any other expectant mother, the thoughts of having a child encompassed my mind most of the day, nearly every day throughout my entire pregnancy. I imagined what it would be like to have a precious newborn in my life and envisioned myself rejoicing in his presence. I did not think about the unexpected turns that would be ever-present in my life once my baby was born. Instead, I thought about meeting my baby for the first time and how life as I knew it would change forever once he or she arrived (we wanted the gender to be a surprise).

Anyone who has ever had a baby knows that the second you tell people you are pregnant, the advice-givers come out of the woodwork. Family, friends, coworkers, neighbors, friends of neighbors, friends of friends of neighbors, even people you meet on the street, all have a story to tell and advice to offer.

Like most first-time mothers, I received an avalanche of advice: how to care for my child, tips on feeding, sleeping, bonding, etc.

Perhaps my uncertainties led me to enjoy receiving these parenting tips. I tried to process all of the advice that was given to me to the best of my abilities; all the while looking forward to seeing my feet again. But in the midst of all of the advice being thrown my way, no one mentioned colic. It wasn't referenced in a single book I received on raising my newborn. Nothing could have been further from my life during my pregnancy. And nothing was more present after my baby's birth.

Tyler was born in the middle of the night after twenty-two hours of intensive labor, followed by a C-section—talk about the unexpected. Despite the physical discomfort and emotional exhaustion of labor and delivery, not once did I think of the whole process as negative. It was a time of pure excitement and joy for me. This was in stark contrast to my experience with having a colicky infant.

Tyler's first cries were truly joyful to me, as I knew he was healthy and trying to communicate his hunger and recognition of the strange new world around him. His second, third, and successive bursts of tears, however, were a little more problematic. There was no pattern to his crying bouts. They arrived in a continuous nature with an increase in their volume and intensity. I had been a parent for less than thirty-six hours, and I had nothing but doubts, anxieties, and real fear. I instinctively knew that something was wrong with my baby because no matter what I tried, no matter what tactics I pursued, Tyler did not stop crying.

At first, I attributed his crying to my own naiveté and inexperience and sought the outside help of nurses, doctors, and lactation specialists. My husband and I attempted to gain as much knowledge and support from those around us as possible. Unfortunately, we soon came to learn that even individuals with an expertise in pediatric medicine could not answer our questions. We expanded our search for answers by eliciting suggestions from people outside the medical profession. We consulted with mental health providers, neighbors, friends, and family—anyone who might provide us with some sort of helpful information to stop the incessant crying.

After only two weeks as a parent, I came to a daunting realization: Tyler's day would be spent screaming and crying while mine would be a spiral of utter despair in not knowing how to help him. In my search to find answers, I came across various definitions and theories of colic. I discovered that (1) there is not any one clear cause of colic specified by doctors, (2) many different theories are cited by many different doctors, some of which contradict one another, and (3) with every theory cited comes few or no answers.

The most popular response to "How do you treat colic?" is time. Researching a condition about which little is known can be frustrating. Doing it while you are sleep deprived, frustrated, confused, and listening to your child's ear-shattering screaming is overwhelmingly depressing. However, as a mother in the midst of trying to handle the devastation of colic and a stubborn clinical psychologist who believes in the idea of problem solving, I chose not to accept the popular response to wait it out and continued on my journey to find some relief. I share my journey here in the hopes of helping others.

How to Use This Book

If you are interested in this book, you are most likely a parent with an infant who won't stop crying and are looking for clear and concrete examples of what you can do to soothe your inconsolable baby. You may also be a person who knows of someone else who is struggling with this problem and would love to help them find some immediate relief. In either case, the information in this book will provide a list of helpful and hopeful interventions that parents can utilize in an attempt to minimize their baby's distress—and at the same time, maintain their own sanity.

In order to provide you with a quick reference of important information and helpful interventions, at the end of each chapter is a review section. This review section is a quick reference guide to the things discussed in that particular chapter. It will provide you with a summary of potential solutions and points of reference to further explore. Remember, every baby is different and what may be causing colic symptoms in one newborn may not be causing colic symptoms in another. I realize that this simple fact in and of itself can lead to frustration while you are looking for answers for your child. I know that it did for me during my long and tedious search for a cure. However, the good news is that there are some tangible answers to your very important questions.

I also realize that due to the urgency of the situation of colic, many of you may be tempted to turn to the end of each chapter and focus solely on the review sections for answers. Believe me when I say that I understand the urgency of finding solutions when you have a colicky infant. However, I will caution you against doing this because the sole purpose of the review sections are to highlight, not detail, information pertaining to assessment, diagnosis, and treatment. Without the detailed information provided in each chapter, you will lose a more thorough account of cause, effect, and intervention strategies. If you are someone who is *desperately* seeking a cure, my recommendation to you is to look at the review section first and then go back to the detailed content in the chapter as a whole in order to gain further knowledge on a particular topic of interest or demand.

A Note from the Author

It is my hope that upon the completion of this book, you will feel both prepared and confident in handling the unexpected challenges that a colicky infant can present. In the midst of exploring the world of colic, this book chronicles a journey of my family's struggles and triumphs in assessing, diagnosing, and treating the problem. As you will see, it depicts how my husband and I aspired to revel in the simple joys of parenthood, but faced the unexpected challenges that a colicky infant presents.

Our family's attempts at finding a solution compelled me to share my experiences with others. However, I want to again acknowledge that every child and family situation is different. I would never suggest that this book unlocks all the mysteries and manifestations of raising a colicky infant. As you will discover, colic did frequently break my spirit as I lost nearly all of the daily battles it presented.

On the other hand, I did manage to win the metaphorical war through perseverance, family support, and the timely discovery of substantive information along the way. It is my sincere hope that *When Your Baby Won't Stop Crying* will increase the knowledge base about colic while emboldening parents that they, too, can survive an infant's colicky period.

Chapter 1

Theories of Colic

O ne of the first things that I was taught in my doctoral training as a clinical psychologist is how to diagnose a problem. However, identifying a problem and giving it a label does not necessarily lead to a cure. Colic is a good example of this. Interestingly, the reason colic is hard to treat has nothing to do with your ability to diagnose it. As you will see, colic is actually not that difficult to diagnose. Instead, the reason colic is hard to treat has more to do with the difficulty in identifying its cause.

In most cases, in order for a doctor to formulate a sound and successful treatment plan, he or she must first identify the cause of the problem. A problem is much harder to treat without this information. For example, think about a person who is running a very high fever. Certainly, a high fever can be a problem and should be treated immediately so the person does not face dire medical consequences. Diagnosing the high fever was probably not a difficult task. A thermometer—or even less scientific, a mother's hand on a child's head—

could reveal a significant rise in body temperature. However, identifying the cause of the high fever may provide doctors with more of a challenge. Many different things could cause a rise in body temperature, for example, an infection, a drug overdose, or heat stroke. The treatment approach for all of these clearly would be very different. Therefore, knowing specifically what the root of the problem is, will allow the doctor to set up a sound treatment plan with hopes for greater success.

In my professional experience, I have found that one of the most common reasons that a treatment plan fails is because the cause has been wrongly determined or not determined at all. Colic is no different. Doctors will often diagnose colic, but have little information as to how to treat it. In order to successfully treat a problem, we must be knowledgeable about the specific causes. With this understanding, we can then begin to formulate our own plan and approach the problem of colic from a more scientific viewpoint.

Background

Colic is diagnosed by the "Rule of Threes"—if an infant cries at least three hours a day, three days per week, for three weeks in a row, then he or she is considered to be suffering from colic.

Much of the current literature states that there is no known cure for colic (with the recent exception of the newborn suffering from gastrointestinal problems). Colic is compared to a virus as experts everywhere attest that colic simply needs to run its course. Colic usually starts when the baby is two weeks old and ends when the baby is one hundred days old, which is approximately three and a half months of age. Some researchers note that colic peaks at six weeks and then begins to dissipate. Interestingly, babies born prematurely usually develop colic two weeks after their original due date and not two weeks after they are born. In addition, premature babies are no more likely to develop colic than a baby who is born at full term.

The sound of the cry of a colicky baby is much more intense than that of other infants. A colicky cry is often described as a piercing, relentless scream. It can stop as abruptly as it starts and is often heard during or immediately after a feeding, especially in cases when it is due to a gastrointestinal problem. The colicky baby sounds as though he is in tremendous pain. His face may be twisted and strained, causing onlookers to be highly concerned. It is not uncommon for concerned parents to show up at emergency rooms in the middle of the night with their colicky infants. If the colic symptoms are caused by gastrointestinal problems, signs of relief may not be apparent until after the infant passes gas or has a bowel movement.

Although there is no known cure for colic, it can be improved with soothing techniques such as offering the baby something to suck on, singing, holding, rocking, white noise, and massage. Colic seems to be much worse at night and during the evening hours, which are often described as the *witching hours*. Many parents complain that this is their infant's fussiest time of day.

Prevalence and Patterns

In the United States, there are approximately four million babies born each year. Each year an estimated one million newborns develop colicky symptoms. That is one out of every four babies! This number may surprise you. I know it left me with two burning questions. First, how could so many families be faced with this hardship and yet so little information on the subject be offered in support of those who endure it? Second, why is a detailed discussion avoided by parents, doctors, child care providers, family, and friends? (See the following discussion on emotional repercussions.)

There is no pattern cited to predict the development of colic. The baby's gender, birth order, or premature status does not predict the onset of colic. In addition, the parents' socioeconomic status, age, education level, or academic achievement has not been linked to colic in any way. Interestingly, not every culture reports colicky infants. In many cultures around the world, babies never get colic.

Many parents proclaim that they believe colic is hereditary. These parents state that they were reportedly colicky infants themselves and that in turn they were "being paid back" with their own colicky infant to raise. There clearly is some validity to this belief. I do not believe it is coincidental that many parents who were colicky themselves have colicky infants.

My husband, Jason, was a colicky infant and so was his father. Tyler was the next to follow in this intergenerational pattern. With the exception once again of gastrointestinal problems, which stem from a biological underpinning, I do not believe that the intergenerational pattern of colic comes from biological or environmental forces. Instead, I believe this link presents itself in the form of personality traits (specifically temperament) and psychological forces (more on this later).

Causes of Colic

There are many theories regarding the various causes of colic. Theories from ancient times include a trauma from pregnancy, the baby catching a draft, the mother's milk being too thin or too rich, and various spiritual and religious beliefs, including possession by the devil and punishment for Adam and Eve's original sin.

There are four frequently cited theories on colic in the current literature. The first and most common is the theory of stomach problems. Gas, constipation, and overactive intestines are cited most frequently in the literature as the causes of colic. This is understandable considering the fact that all three of these factors can unquestionably lead to a feeling of discomfort, causing a baby to cry. In fact, the word colic is derived from a Greek word, *kolikos*, which means "large intestine or colon." In the past, parents believed that stomach pain and/or discomfort caused their babies to cry. This theory has definitely stuck through the years.

When Jason and I informed people that Tyler was colicky, the most common initial response was "Colic—that's when a baby cries all the time, right?" Then the second response would be "Isn't it because of gas or stomach problems?" Doctors, family, and friends are quick to assume that these "tummy troubles" (as they are often referred to in the literature) are the main reason for the colicky infant's relentless crying. Although all of these factors can potentially cause a baby to cry, there are several reasons why I came to believe that they are not the only or main cause of colic.

Two different types of stomach problems are cited in the literature. One is much more severe than the other. The less severe problem is characterized by great discomfort due to problems with the baby's digestive system. An infant's digestive system is not fully mature until he or she is one hundred days old. Therefore, gas, constipation, and stomach cramps may cause such great distress that the infant cries out in pain. The more severe problem is characterized by severe abdominal pain due to intestinal illness, such as stomach acid reflux or food intolerance/allergy. The good news is that newborns who have this medical problem can be medically treated. In other words, under this specific circumstance, there is a cure.

Infants who are suffering from gastroesophageal reflux disease (also known as infant GERD) can be treated with certain medications. These medications must be prescribed by a medical doctor. Please consult your pediatrician immediately if you believe your newborn may be suffering from this problem. (See Chapter 4, "Treatment Approaches for Specific Causes," for a more detailed account of gassiness and infant GERD and tips on how to combat this problem.)

Infants who are suffering from food intolerance/allergy may also find a cure. However, some detective work may be necessary. When a newborn has a food intolerance/allergy, the caregiver must first find the cause of the problem in order to find the cure. Once the food or ingredient causing the problem is found, then it can be avoided to provide the infant with some relief. (See Chapter 4, "Treatment Approaches for Specific Causes," for a more detailed account of possible food intolerances/allergies and tips on how to combat this problem.)

The second highly cited theory involves brain development. This theory states that when a baby's nervous system is not fully matured, it can cause the baby to feel overwhelmed and as a result the baby will cry. I was thoroughly intrigued by this theory. It made a lot of sense to me. Babies have been in the womb for nine months with minimal stimulation. Once born, they are faced with new sounds, smells, sights, and touch. I could only imagine how overstimulating this could be for a newborn.

I was hesitant to accept this theory as a whole because only some infants are colicky. If this theory were true, wouldn't all infants be colicky? What was the deciding factor? Were the brains of colicky infants less mature than other infant brains or was something missing in this theory? I decided that something must be missing. I based this decision on one important fact. The most immature brain is found in a baby born prematurely. However, premature babies are no more likely than full-term babies to develop colic.

The third theory focuses on maternal anxiety. It states that mothers who are anxious elicit the same anxious response in their babies. In other words, the anxious mother transfers her anxieties onto her infant, which in turn causes the infant to cry. To be honest, I am not a particular fan of this theory, and many parents agree. After all, this theory blames the mother for her baby's colic. Many parents find this theory upsetting to read about. It is the one theory that feeds right into the mother of a colicky infant's already existing insecurities. Initially, most mothers do not want to accept this theory because accepting it means they are fully to blame.

From working for so many years in the field of psychology, I have become all too familiar with blame being placed on parents or on a victim. In fact, one of the easiest theories to develop is a theory of blame. However, it was the first time that I was actually in that hot seat. It did not feel good to be blamed for my child's problems. As a parent with a colicky infant, I felt victimized by my circumstances. In a sense, parents are victims of this traumatic experience. Colic can be extremely traumatizing for the entire family unit, not just the infant. In turn, the last thing a new mother needs or wants to think about is being the cause of this terrible situation. However, this theory suggests just that: a mother who is anxious may be causing colic.

In an attempt to investigate this possibility, I made a conscious effort to place my insecurities aside and to look at this theory logically to decide whether or not it had some credibility. I was a new mother who did not feel fully equipped to handle all of the challenges that came along with motherhood. Caring for a newborn can be unexpectedly stressful for first-time mothers. It is a life-altering circumstance.

While researching the validity of this theory, I reminded myself of the reasons for a mother's stress. The instability of hormones, sleep deprivation, and bodily changes combined frequently with a loss of financial income and professional gratification, plus isolation from friends, coworkers, and family members can all cause tremendous amounts of tension and pressure in the mother's life. (See Chapter 7, "Taking Care of the Caretaker," for quick tips on how to support the new mother.)

Research does indicate that stress and anxiety can affect both biological and psychological processes in the new mother. For example, biologically, stress can lessen the mother's milk supply or interfere with proper letdown. If this occurs, the infant can become hungry and cry. Psychologically, stress can cause the mother to become increasingly distracted, perhaps avoiding attending to and handling her infant. One doctor who specializes in soothing techniques for colicky infants notes that anxious mothers tend to jump from one soothing technique to another, which can potentially upset a baby more and have the opposite of the desired effect.

With all of the research on anxious mothers, it is hard to deny that this does not play some role in the potential for a colicky infant. However, I strongly believe that this is not a sole cause of colic. I have seen plenty of mothers both personally and professionally who have extreme anxiety both during and after pregnancy but have calm, peaceful infants who cry minimally in their first months of life. Also, let's not forget, there is no link between colic and birth order. Colic can occur with a firstborn as likely as it can occur with a sixth born. Therefore, wouldn't we expect more experienced parents to be more confident and less anxious? But they could still have a colicky infant.

The last current theory that is cited in colic literature focuses on the baby's temperament. Sensitive babies will inevitable respond more intensely to things that cause them distress and as a result get upset and cry more. Most researchers believe, and many parents agree, that a baby is born with a certain temperament. I hear mothers talk all the time about knowing exactly what type of child they will have according to the activity in the womb. Many people believe it starts that early, and most concur that it is present at birth. In addition, it is argued that one's temperament is a stable trait, which means it usually will not change throughout one's lifetime.

After reading this theory, I thought about Tyler's temperament and whether there were any clues during pregnancy about his sensitive nature. There were some. The two that I remember most clearly had to do with his intense reactions to taste and sound. I remembered that when I ate spicy food, Tyler would do somersaults in utero. Toward the end of my pregnancy he would hiccup after every large meal I ate. He was sensitive both to the types of food I ate and the quantity of food that I consumed.

Tyler was also sensitive to sound when *in utero*. He would respond with very strong kicks to any loud noises around him. Jason and I rented a Doppler machine so that we could listen to his heartbeat whenever we wanted to during pregnancy. As Tyler grew bigger and there was less room for him to move around in utero he became increasingly agitated by the use of this machine. Each time we turned it on, Tyler responded to it. We found it astonishing that he would kick at the machine as if to say, "Shut that thing off!" Suffice it to say, we sent it back early, but we were amazed at his sensitive response to sound (not to mention the precision in his kicks—an athlete in the making, I was sure).

Since colicky babies clearly can be sensitive in nature and respond to stimuli in intense ways (their relentless screaming), I believe this theory has some credibility. However, I am not fully convinced that this alone causes colic. I can think of at least three of my friends who had particularly sensitive children, and not one of them suffered from colic as infants.

After researching the current theories on colic, I was faced with the realization and confirmation that there probably was not one sole cause of colic—unless the infant was struggling from one of the stomach illnesses listed above. I came to develop a theory on colic that made sense to me (see Chapter 5, "Finally an Answer") by combining information from many of the different theories listed above as well as from the detective work that my family did in order to find some relief.

Emotional Repercussions

I will refer to the trauma or the traumatic nature of colic on the entire family system in several places throughout this book. The emotional repercussions due to colic can be devastating for all family members involved. I think it is fair to say that for most caregivers, first and foremost they are concerned for their infant's well-being. I believe that instinctively the majority of parents want to protect and care for their children. In my office, parents often tell me, "If I could take my child's pain away, I would." Their desire to help and their motivation to protect their babies from harm is heartwarming.

This situation is often no different for parents with a colicky infant. However, the issue of physical pain needs to be addressed because many experts believe that the colicky infant is not experiencing pain (unless the colic is due to a gastrointestinal problem). In fact, most doctors agree that the infant does not feel pain at all during a colicky episode, and perhaps more important, doctors agree that the distress the infant does feel will not be remembered by him later in life. When I told Tyler's pediatrician, who had a colicky infant of her own, "I feel so bad for him; it breaks my heart that I cannot get him to stop crying," her response to me was, "I feel bad for *you!*" She went on to say, "He won't remember any of this when he gets older, but unfortunately, you will never forget it!"

It is important to recognize that the degree of severity of colic symptoms is variable. Thus, in turn, the level of traumatization produced by the colicky symptoms will also vary. Perhaps this is one of the reasons that it is not addressed among sufferers. Still, the feelings of insecurity, fear, frustration, and resentment can be overwhelming and should not be ignored.

There were days I felt so distraught and on edge I could actually understand how individuals could harm their children. I never acted on these thoughts, but they were definitely there during the tougher times.

It seems that only the stories of the unstable individuals who do harm their children due to their intense feelings of hopelessness and helplessness come to the media's attention and in turn become the topic of conversation in the average household. We gasp at the horror of the unthinkable—harming a poor defenseless child. However, understanding what drives a person to do the unthinkable is never addressed.

It is difficult for individuals to reach out for help if they know that they will be criticized, judged, and shunned for doing so. That is not to say that fear of criticism or judgment is an excuse for non-solicitation, but it can be described as a deterrent and unfortunately without some form of support in those special circumstances, the consequences for the baby can be dire.

Clearly, most parents with colicky infants do not harm their children in any way. However, I cannot help but wonder if many of the babies who are victims of abuse suffer from colic. If you are skeptical about this proposition, think about this: the most common answer among perpetrators of infant abuse (including perpetrators of shaken baby syndrome) is "My baby would not stop crying!"

I remember some of my friends, who had heard through the grapevine that Tyler was colicky, told us that they would be willing to come over and baby-sit any time to help out. It's a funny thing when you have a colicky infant. You do not seem to enlist help from others as you would if your child was not colicky. I think there are several reasons for this, including: (1) embarrassment, (2) fear, and (3) concern. As a stable parent, it was hard to handle all of the relentless crying. How could I inflict it on someone else? Moreover, how could I be sure they, who didn't necessarily love this baby the way I do, wouldn't succumb to frustrations themselves, with dire consequences.

CHAPTER REVIEW

Assessment and Diagnosis of Colic

Dr. Wessel's "Rule of Threes"
If an infant cries at least three hours a day, three days per week, for three weeks in a row, then he or she is considered to be suffering from colic.

Colic's Course
Colic usually starts when the baby is two weeks old and ends when the baby is one hundred days old (approximately three and a half months of age). Colic often peaks at six weeks and then begins to dissipate.

Parent Observation
The sound of the colic cry is intense—often described as a piercing, relentless scream. It can stop as abruptly as it starts and is often heard during or immediately after a feeding (when it is due to a gastrointestinal problem). The baby's face may be twisted and strained, causing onlookers to be highly concerned.

Witching Hours
Often worse at night, bouts of crying in the evening hours are often described as the witching hours.

Prevalence and Patterns
* In the United States, 20 to 25 percent of infants suffer from colic.
* There is no pattern cited to predict the development of colic.
* Many parents believe colic is hereditary.

* I believe the hereditary link of colic presents itself in the form of personality traits (specifically temperament) and psychological forces.

Causes of Colic

Theory of Stomach Problems
Gas, constipation, and overactive intestines are cited most frequently in the literature as the cause of colic.

Two types: problems with the baby's immature digestive system or intestinal illness, such as stomach acid reflux or food intolerance/allergy.

Brain Development
This theory states that when a baby's nervous system is not fully matured, it can cause the baby to feel overwhelmed, and as a result the baby cries.

Maternal Anxiety
Mothers who are anxious elicit the same anxious response in their babies.

Baby's Temperament
Sensitive babies will inevitably respond more intensely to things that cause them distress, and as a result get upset and cry more.

Emotional Repercussions for the Parent
* Feelings of hopelessness and helplessness, and feeling overwhelmed.
* Thoughts of being a "bad parent."
* Fear of judgment and/or criticism by others.
* Isolation due to all of the above.

Chapter 2

The First Sign of Trouble

Assessing a problem is the very first step in finding a solution. The sooner you can identify that there is a problem, the sooner you can attempt to solve it. In the case of colic specifically, the earlier you are able to recognize that your baby is exhibiting these symptoms, the sooner you can gain an understanding of the problem and search for a cause. Once a cause is found, you will be better equipped to utilize strategies that will provide both you and your baby with some relief.

Although many babies do not manifest signs of colic until two weeks of age, in my son's case, onset of colicky symptoms was very shortly after birth.

My Story: The Onset of Colic

After twenty-two hours of labor followed by a C-section, I was both physically and emotionally exhausted. When I felt my first contraction early that memorable morning, I had no idea that late the next evening

I would be recovering from a major surgery. Yet none of this seemed to matter because I was finally able to hold my firstborn son in my arms.

It was my first time staying overnight in a hospital. I was very lucky in my life—I'd never broken a bone, required surgery, or experienced a severe illness leading to a prolonged hospital stay. I knew I would not want to be in the hospital longer than necessary, so Jason and I opted to leave one day earlier than the allotted time for a C-section birth. In retrospect, I wish I had stayed the full time permitted. I had no idea what I was about to be confronted with in its most severe and intense form: colic. Dealing with a colicky infant for the next six months was the furthest thing from my mind.

My husband stayed with me in the hospital. Neither one of us had any family in the area, so our close friends came to visit us soon after the birth to share in our excitement and joy. It was a wonderful feeling introducing people to our most precious baby boy. We realized how blessed we were to have such a wonderful support system around us, since most of our family was thousands of miles away. My mother was scheduled to fly out to visit and help me upon my arrival home. We spent only one night alone in our house before she arrived.

The day before we went home, Jason left the hospital to check in on our house and our dog. Jason wanted to take a shower and prepare the house for our arrival the following day. He was gone from the hospital for approximately three hours. This may sound like a very short amount of time, but what occurred in his absence made it feel as though it was a lifetime.

Tyler woke up from a nap and was hungry. I was beginning to get the breast-feeding thing, but my milk had not come in yet, so Tyler was still feeding off of colostrum. The mechanics of breast-feeding were becoming easier, but the process was still a struggle because I knew he was not getting enough of what he needed. After he was fed, he began to cry. At first, I was not concerned. I was already accustomed to hearing him cry and usually was able to figure out what was bothering him. I figured he was hungry, wet, tired, or uncomfortable. I checked his diaper and he was dry. I held him in my arms, rocking him slowly back and forth. I sang to him softly in his ear. I even tried burping him again in case he had some extra gas from the feeding. Nothing seemed to help.

Tyler's cries seemed to grow louder and louder. I was becoming worried that something might be wrong and called for a nurse. She checked on him for me and found that he was perfectly healthy, and said he was, "Probably just tired or having a newborn moment." I decided to take him for a walk around the hospital ward. However, his incessant screaming became so loud, I was afraid it would wake up all of the other babies and parents trying to get some rest from their own labors and deliveries.

Singing, swaying, and shushing in the cramped quarters of my hospital room while my three-day-old son was relentlessly screaming his head off began to make me wonder if I knew what I was doing. I couldn't wait for Jason to get back to the hospital. I was wishing he never left. Unfortunately, the hospital wall clock revealed that he had only been gone for one hour.

After another thirty minutes of continuous crying, I called Jason at home and I told him I needed him to come back to the hospital as fast as he could. I did not admit it to him at the time, but I was scared. All of a sudden I was feeling very much alone. Tyler would not stop crying and there was nothing I could do about it.

Jason finally made it back to the hospital. Tyler was still crying when he entered the room. He looked surprised. Tyler had worked himself up into quite a frenzy by this point. Jason immediately asked what was wrong. He and I had never seen the baby this upset before. However, we also had never had a baby before and Tyler was only three days old. Our experience started and ended with him. We had no idea what was normal and what was not, but we both instinctively knew something was very wrong.

Jason left to go get a nurse. She came into the room, picked Tyler up, and then re-swaddled him. He fell right to sleep. Jason and I looked at each other and then at her. We were embarrassed by the notion that we had absolutely no idea of what we were doing. The nurse politely supported our efforts as she left the room.

Once alone, I told Jason about the horrible three hours I had with Tyler screaming nonstop. I was glad Tyler was finally asleep. Both Jason and I were exhausted. I did not realize how emotionally and physically draining those first few days would be, and we had the support of a whole hospital staff. The nurses came in to help with everything. If I was sleeping, they woke me up every couple of hours to make sure Tyler breast-fed. They brought food, water, pillows, and anything else we asked for to make the stay more comfortable and less overwhelming. I wondered how in the world I would do this all on my own.

When Tyler woke up from his nap, he immediately started crying again. It was 6:00 p.m. He did not sleep for very long; one hour at the most. I assumed after three consecutive hours of crying, he would be exhausted and would sleep a little longer, but what did I know? I was a new mom with absolutely no experience, and let's face it; this little three-day-old baby was wearing me down.

I decided to try breast-feeding him again, thinking he might be hungry. I knew I was. I had not eaten all day. I was still on a special diet following my surgery. Luckily, Tyler latched on easily, ate well, and calmed down immediately. Jason and I watched him as he ate. He was so tiny. We were in awe that we created such a perfect little being.

I finished breast-feeding Tyler and handed him to Jason, who held him for less than a minute when the crying started again. Jason changed his diaper and tried to swaddle him the way the nurse did earlier to give him more security and comfort. However, our swaddling technique was far from perfected at this point. After three tries, we called the nurse back into our room embarrassed once again by our ineptness. She showed us how to swaddle our baby correctly, but this time Tyler continued to cry. The nurse suggested that I breast-feed again.

I tried to breast-feed Tyler for the second time in one hour, but he would not latch onto my breast. Each time I tried to help him, he screamed louder. Why was this not working? I could feel the tears welling up in my eyes. I was becoming frustrated and I was thoroughly exhausted. The nurse came back into the room and tried to help me. Upon seeing that Tyler was refusing the breast, she asked if she could try a bottle. I burst into tears. As strange as it may sound, I think introducing the bottle somehow symbolized a failure to me. I am used to feeling in control and helping others. As a clinical psychologist, it is my job to help others and I am usually successful in doing so. However, in this situation, I could not help, I could not control, I could not make things better. My efforts were fruitless and I knew it. It was a terrible feeling. I was on an emotional roller coaster ride. My hormones were raging, and I was clearly tired, frustrated, and confused. I was also feeling overwhelmed, scared, and helpless.

Jason immediately came to my side to comfort me. All I could do was cry. As irrational as it may have been, I felt the sadness in my heart. After a few moments had passed, I told the nurse we could try the bottle. In order to entice Tyler to latch onto my breast, she provided us with a very helpful tip. She squeezed some formula out of the bottle onto my nipple. It worked. Tyler stopped crying and started breast-feeding on his own.

After Tyler finished feeding, he seemed content. However, by this time even Jason was starting to look exhausted. The nurse asked us if we wanted to have Tyler sleep in the nursery that night. As tempting as it sounded, Jason and I made a firm decision before entering the hospital that we would not leave Tyler for a minute once he was born. Therefore, we declined her offer.

The hospital provided a bassinet in our room so that we would not have to be separated from our baby. This really appealed to us. Why is it that no matter how uncommon it may be, it is the horror stories about babies being switched at birth, stolen, or accidentally dropped out of their bassinets that people remember the most? Jason and I were not going to take any chances. Tyler would sleep with us every night—or so we thought.

Approximately one hour after Tyler's feeding, he was crying again. I reached over and picked him up. As I rocked him in my arms, his cries became louder. Jason woke up and tried to help. He walked Tyler around the room as I prepared to breast-feed. Tyler ate and then cried some more. He was burped and then cried some more. He was changed and then cried some more. He was swaddled and then cried some more. He was rocked—still crying. He was walked around the room again—still crying. He was sung to—still crying. He was gently shushed—still crying. The nurse came in to help—he was still crying. He was healthy and medically stable—and still crying. I am sure by now you are getting the point.

Two and a half hours later, Tyler finally fell asleep. The hospital was quiet. Jason suggested that we allow the nurse to bring Tyler to the nursery so we could get some sleep. Forget our earlier decision— we were tired. We prayed there would still be some room for him. We prayed they would take him, temperament and all. They did, and we finally slept.

At 3:00 a.m. Tyler was brought to me for a middle of the night feeding. He ate well and fell back asleep—thank God. At 6:00 a.m. Tyler was brought for an early-morning feeding. He ate well and fell back asleep—thank God. At 9:00 a.m. Tyler was brought to me for a late-morning feeding. He ate well and fell back asleep—thank God. Jason and I slept as best we could with all the interruptions and were surprised at how quickly daylight came.

That morning Jason and I planned to take Tyler home. We struggled to put him in his car seat, but managed it. Jason commented that it was surprising how easily new parents are seen off with a wave, a "good luck," and a small parent blue book—everything you need to know in five simple pages. That's it! We left without a clue of what to do next.

We arrived home and talked about how strange it was to actually have a son. As unreal as it may have felt, at least we knew we were prepared. We spent months preparing for the moment we would bring our child home. The nursery had been finished in every miniscule detail. Diapers and wipes were bought; clothes were stacked neatly in the dresser drawers; breast pumps and bottles were laid out on the kitchen table ready to be used as needed. We purchased a glider chair and a Boppy to make breast-feeding easier and more comfortable. We had a small bassinet positioned next to our bed where Tyler would sleep the first few weeks before moving into his own bedroom. Everything was available, ready, and waiting for use.

Our first night at home was not much different from our hospital stay. Tyler woke up every few hours for his feeding. He was changed a few times and burped and then fell back asleep. My milk still had not yet come in, and I was becoming a little worried. He had lost nearly a pound by the time we left the hospital. I was told that was not uncommon, but I did not want him to lose any more weight while he was at home. I was hoping that my milk would come in by the following day.

The next day my mother arrived. I could not wait to see her and introduce her to her first grandchild. We all went to pick her up at the airport. I could see her standing out front waiting for us. I will never forget the look on her face as she peered through the car window at her first grandchild. She was standing on the curb holding her travel bag and watching Tyler sleep like a little angel. It was a memorable moment, one of the few I would be able to reflect upon without the inclusion of colicky cries.

Our drive home from the airport went quickly. We talked about our experience with labor and delivery and our hospital stay thereafter. Tyler woke up just as we pulled into the driveway. He started to cry as we went inside the house. My mother took him out of the car seat and held him for the first time. I remember watching her hold him with such grace, confidence, and ease—something else Jason and I had not perfected yet. She made it look so simple. We were both still afraid that if we handled him incorrectly he would break.

I breast-fed Tyler on the couch as we visited. I was beginning to get used to the fact that we actually had a living, breathing child in our home. I think it really hit me for the first time when I sat with my mother and my baby at the same time.

At 8:00 p.m. that night Tyler fell asleep. Since he was only a few days old, he had not yet established any type of sleeping pattern. We all figured we should sleep while we could because nobody really knew when he would wake up next. I knew I would be up to feed him in a few hours and wanted to get to bed right away.

At 10:00 p.m. Tyler woke up crying in his bassinet. I picked him up and cradled him in my arms. His cry seemed different to me than others I had heard before, but I was a new mom and really did not think much about this at the time. I checked his diaper, found that he was wet, and changed him. I carried him over to the glider chair where I breast-fed him. Tyler was still crying, but his cries were becoming louder and more intense. I remember thinking, "Boy, he must really be hungry." I quickly got into position for his feeding and tried to get him to latch onto the breast, but he refused. I was surprised. This had never happened before (at least not when he was hungry), and to be honest, I had no idea what to do about it. His cries were rapidly growing in volume and intensity. I knew if I did not do something fast, the whole house would awaken. I tried to soothe him by singing to him and telling him it would be okay while trying to get him to latch onto my breast.

At that moment, Jason and my mother walked into the nursery asking what was wrong. I explained the situation and they tried to help, but Tyler wouldn't budge. This was definitely not something they prepared us for at the hospital. Jason took Tyler and tried to soothe him by rocking him in his arms. He only cried more. My mother took a turn and tried to soothe him by singing gently in his ear while walking him around the house. He still cried. I tried to breast-feed him again to no avail. He cried and cried!

We were all beginning to get a little worried. I looked to my mother for answers. My mother seemed as confused by the crying as we were. We passed Tyler around to one another several times trying different tactics to soothe him (burping, singing, rocking, walking, swaying, etc.). Finally, after about an hour of crying, he settled down and latched onto my breast. We were all exhausted. It is incredible how emotionally draining it can be with an infant, especially your own child, while he or she is crying. The feelings of helplessness were unbearable! One hour felt like eight hours.

I stayed with Tyler for forty minutes while he fed on both breasts consecutively. He fell asleep on the second breast, and instead of putting him in his crib immediately, I stayed with him for a while to watch him sleep. He looked so peaceful. How could an infant go from such anguish to such peace in only a matter of minutes? After approximately fifteen minutes, I gently pulled him off my breast and placed him back in his crib. He was already wrapped in his blanket and ready for sleep.

As I got into bed myself, I hoped to get a few hours of restful sleep before the next feeding. However, before my second leg was even in the bed, Tyler started crying again. His cries sounded similar to the cries heard just moments before. He was clearly distressed about something. I jumped out of bed and went back into the nursery and picked him up. He was not wet and he had just eaten. However, I tried to feed him again out of desperation and uncertainty. My milk had still not come in, so Tyler was still feeding on colostrum. I wondered if he was hungry.

Common Concerns

Parents who are encountering their newborn's relentless cries for the first time face several common fears. One of the most common concerns stated by parents is the fear of their newborn being hungry and not getting enough food. This is particularly scary for parents when the mother's milk has not yet come in. Infants usually lose weight in the first few days of their lives, but gain it back once the mother's milk comes in and they are able to eat larger meals.

I had this fear several times during the first few days of Tyler's life. My milk had not come in yet and I was certain that Tyler was not getting enough food and was hungry. Initially it was hard for me to consider other options, but I did utilize the two options suggested to me by the nurses in the hospital, both of them with varying success.

The first option, dropping some formula onto the nipple in order to entice the baby to breast-feed, worked most of the time, unless

Tyler was in the midst of a colicky crying burst and was not hungry. The second option, bottle-feeding, I had less success with. Tyler was not as comfortable with the bottle and did not take to it easily. In one desperate moment, Jason and I even tried squeezing some out into his mouth to help him understand he would be fed. However, this only seemed to increase his anger and his refusal to eat continued.

Another common concern experienced by parents is the unknown cause of the intense cries. Parents often worry that their newborn is in excruciating pain. They instinctively believe that something is very wrong with their infant and that he should be examined by a doctor. I remember often worrying about this with Tyler before he was diagnosed with colic. His cries were consistent, outrageously loud, and incredibly strong. He often cried for several consecutive hours, growing more and more agitated by the minute.

It is not uncommon for parents to rush their baby to an emergency room in fear that he is going to hurt himself, pop a blood vessel, or have a seizure due to his relentless crying. The very first night my mother was in town I asked her if we should take Tyler to the emergency room. I remember that even she was worried. Something seemed to be very wrong with him. It did not seem normal to have a baby cry for several consecutive hours in a row. We decided to wait a little bit longer to see if Tyler would eventually cry himself to sleep.

It is common for babies to cry and it is even more common for them to cry themselves to sleep out of utter exhaustion when left to their own devices. However, this is not true for colicky infants. They tend to wind themselves up instead of wind themselves down. You may have heard parents talk about letting their children cry themselves to sleep at night. This strategy became very well known and even perfected by Dr. Richard Ferber, who invented the Ferber technique in 1985. Richard Ferber is the director of the Center for Pediatric Sleep

Disorders at Children's Hospital in Boston. He is a pediatric sleep expert and the author of *Solve Your Child's Sleep Problems.*

The Ferber technique is based on the premise that you progressively train your baby to fall asleep on his own. At bedtime, the infant is placed in his crib while he is still awake. If he cries, parents wait a certain amount of time before going in and checking on him. If the crying continues, the baby is left alone for increasing amounts of time before the parent comes in to acknowledge him. The check-ins do not entail picking the baby up or feeding him, but rather simply allowing the baby to hear the soothing sound of your voice and only for a short period of time. Dr. Ferber estimates that after approximately one week, the infant learns to sleep on his own because crying only provides him with a brief check-in from his parents.

Even though this strategy is well known and applauded by many, as my son cried relentlessly every night, all I kept wondering was why is this not working? Never did I remember hearing parents talk about it taking hours for their children to cry themselves to sleep. I knew that if I tried this with Tyler, it could take days. Instead of becoming tired and settling down, he was becoming more agitated.

Another common concern often mentioned by parents is that in the midst of a colicky crying episode, their baby does not eat. Some parents note that their baby may not eat for eight straight hours due to a colicky outburst. Tyler was this way. He often refused to eat when crying and frequently would not eat for long periods of time. It was as if his cries were upsetting even to himself and nothing—not even food—would disrupt this pattern. The good news is that babies do not typically starve themselves and will eat when they are hungry enough.

Similar to parents' fear of the baby not receiving enough food is the fear of the baby not receiving enough sleep. In the midst of a colicky crying episode, their baby does not sleep. Sometimes parents note that their baby will catch up on sleep later; however, this is not always the case. Although sleep deprivation is not preferable, doctors confirm that babies will eventually sleep when they become tired enough.

Emerging Emotions in the Assessment Phase

Sometimes it is the most basic and simplest things that cause the parent of a colicky infant to feel angry, sad, or confused. For example, I remember the first night that Tyler cried consistently throughout the night. It was 1:00 a.m. and Jason had to go to work the next morning. He had not been to sleep yet. In the midst of Tyler's cries, my mother convinced him to go to bed and get some sleep. At first he refused. He wanted to stay up and help or at least show his support. However, with her persuasion, he reluctantly complied and went to bed.

It was the first time I felt a tinge of jealously and anger toward him. Why did he get to go to bed? It seemed unfair. I knew these thoughts were childlike. I immediately felt guilty for having them. Although they quickly passed as I held my screaming infant it was clear to me that they were very real and would probably return in the weeks to come.

When you are the parent of a colicky infant there are moments when it seems as if there is no time to feel or to think. Your newborn is relentless. It feels as if you have no control over the situation (at least not in the beginning before you know what to do). These factors can lead a parent to feel utter despair. It can also lead the parent to feel very much alone.

Despair and isolation are two emotions that can be highly detrimental to the psyche. They are clear indicators of depression and high-risk factors for suicidal ideation. If you or someone you know is struggling with these feelings, it is important to seek help. Gaining support and hope is key in getting through these tough times.

A woman once shared a story with me about her darkest hour as a parent. On one very momentous sleep-deprived day, she got into her car and started driving to her daughter's pediatrician. As she arrived in the parking lot, she realized she had left her daughter at home. Luckily, her husband was home and cared for their daughter in her absence.

This woman's daughter was three weeks old when she first showed signs of colic. By the time she was six weeks old, she was crying a minimum of ten hours per day. To make matters worse, this baby was a poor sleeper who did not sleep longer than twenty to thirty minutes at a time. She was also a slow eater, feeding forty minutes on each breast at a given sitting. This woman complained that there was absolutely no time to do anything for her other child, her husband, her home, and probably least important to her, for herself. Her biggest struggle was the lack of sleep that she was getting. She estimated that she was getting a mere three hours of sleep per day.

In addition, her older child was in school every day and her husband was at work with a job that required a lot of travel. With no family in the area, she spent almost every day alone just trying to get by. Her isolation and growing despair quickly led to suicidal thoughts. She stated, "The only thing that kept me from hurting myself was the thought of my kids being without a mother." She knew she had to be there for her family, but did not know how she would get through this difficult time alone. Luckily, her daughter's colic peaked at six weeks and began to diminish. By the time her daughter was three and a half months old, the colic was gone.

I can easily recall one of my darkest moments in the midst of Tyler's colic. He was less than a week old and it was the first time he cried for almost twelve hours straight. I tried everything I could that day and night to soothe him. After nine hours of relentless crying, he finally fell asleep. Holding him in my arms in our backyard while slowly swinging him on our swing set seemed to do the trick. I remember letting him sleep for at least twenty minutes before attempting to get up. I wanted to ensure he was sound asleep and would not wake up. When I reentered the house, the unbelievable happened. Tyler woke up and started crying again. I quickly stepped back outside, but the damage was done. He was awake and angry, and nothing was going to change that. I remember thinking, "Could this really be happening?" I was shocked.

I quickly moved to the far side of our house (which is not very big) to try to shield Jason and my mother from the noise so that they could continue to get some sleep. They had been up with me most of the night. I locked myself in our office, which is located off the garage. This seemed to work as a temporary shield. Both Jason and my mother slept through the next two hours of what I would describe as pure screaming hell. Tyler did not stop crying a single second during that two-hour period.

I felt like crying myself, but I think I was too tired to muster up the energy to shed a tear. I couldn't even think straight. I was surprised how such a small individual could create sounds of such magnitude. However, I was not surprised at Tyler's persistence. Unfortunately this is a gene he inherited from both sides of the gene pool. Both his father and I can be unbelievably stubborn. In addition, Tyler is a Taurus. Need I say more? Nevertheless, the night was heart-wrenching and unbearable.

At 6:00 a.m. I finally was able to get Tyler to eat. He latched onto my breast and nursed for thirty minutes. He fell asleep during his feeding and was finally at peace. I decided to put him in his bassinet and place his bassinet in his larger crib, which was located in the nursery. I did not want to go back into my bedroom with him. I was terrified that he would wake up at any given moment and start crying again. I also didn't want to disturb Jason, who was also sound asleep.

I was able to transition Tyler successfully (without waking him up) into his big crib where he continued to sleep soundly. I laid down on the floor of the nursery next to his crib in anticipation. I covered myself with one of his baby blankets, which covered only a small portion of my body, and waited. I was cold, tired, and hungry, but I did not dare to move. All I could do was cry.

Once I started crying I couldn't stop. I was emotionally devastated and drained. I was scared, overwhelmed, and confused. I was sure to keep my cries soft so that I would not wake up the baby. I laid on the hardwood floor questioning what had just happened for the past ten hours. I thought about the trauma of the long, hard night. I once again doubted myself and my abilities to parent. I remember thinking that I was a terrible mother who couldn't even find a way to comfort her own child. Wasn't this supposed to be instinctual or some sort of innate ability shared by mothers all around the world? Why was I not able to do what seems to come so naturally to so many women? At that moment, I felt extremely alone.

As with the woman whom I described earlier who left her daughter at home, I was both physically and emotionally exhausted. I felt utter despair and isolation. Having two family members in the house did not change that. Luckily, I did receive support from them the next day.

At 7:00 a.m. Jason entered the nursery. He found me on the floor with my face buried in a receiving blanket sobbing quietly. His alarm had gone off at 6:30 a.m. and he got up to get ready for work. I didn't even hear him. He thought I had fallen asleep out on the sofa in the family room and tried to make as little noise as possible so as not to disturb me or the baby. When he woke up, he heard complete silence in the house. Therefore, he assumed that everyone was sleeping soundly.

When Jason entered the nursery, I turned my body away from him. I was embarrassed about my uncontrollable sobbing and did not want him to be concerned about me. Could I possibly expect him to understand the feelings that I was experiencing after that long hard night?

I thought about the difference between women and men, mothers and fathers.

Jason is the most loving, supportive man I have ever known, but he is not a mother. I knew at some level he might understand, but he would have a different perspective on the situation than I. To be honest, at that moment I did not have the energy to try to explain my feelings or my perspective to him. I barely understood them myself and I was completely exhausted, so I turned away. This act was not out of anger or resentment, but rather as a means of self-preservation.

Perhaps the many years that Jason has been married to a psychologist who strongly believes in verbal self-expression and open communication paid off in my time of despair. That morning he instinctively knew something was wrong. He bent down on one knee and began stroking my hair as I laid on the floor. At first he did not say a word. He simply sat with me and allowed me to feel his physical presence. It was extremely comforting. He then leaned over and kissed me on the head and whispered into my ear, "Are you okay?" I could tell he was confused as to what was happening, and that he was concerned about my well-being.

That morning, I did not need to respond to Jason's question, because he knew the answer. I was not okay. He didn't push for answers to his questions about what occurred that night that left his wife in such a traumatized state. I was grateful for this because I could not speak nor did I want to. I could only lie there on the floor and cry. Jason decided to lie down on the floor next to me. He held me tightly in his arms. He continued to stroke my hair and comfort me with his actions. I could hear his silent concern and felt his love and care for me.

How to Help

In an attempt to support someone who is struggling with a colicky infant, the first and most important thing to remember is that she is on an emotional roller-coaster ride. Encourage the person to verbalize her feelings, but do not pressure her to talk before she is ready. Utilize active listening skills when she does begin to share her struggles and distressing emotions. Do not judge or criticize her feelings. Do not tell her not to feel that way. Do not minimize the way she is feeling or tell her that she is only trying to get attention.

CHAPTER REVIEW

What to Look For
* The infant cries for more than three consecutive hours per day.
* The infant cries are loud, intense, and relentless.
* The infant does not easily cry himself to sleep.
* The infant is frequently disinterested in eating during crying bouts. Thus, the baby is not crying because he is hungry.
* The infant is inconsolable.

Common Concerns and What to Know
* There may be some breaks in crying due to the utilization of distraction or soothing techniques.
* It is not uncommon for parents to worry that their baby may hurt himself due to the intensity of his colicky cries.
* Due to the continuous, inconsolable nature of the child's distress, parents often experience their own distress.

Emerging Emotions
* Feelings of confusion, shock, fear, anxiety, anger, helplessness, and hopelessness are common among parents during the assessment phase and thereafter.
* During the initial assessment phase, both emotional and physical exhaustion is common among parents.
* Parent adjustment to colicky symptoms occurs later.
* Support of the parent is particularly important during this phase.

Chapter 3

Diagnosing the Problem

As I have mentioned before, diagnosing colic is not that difficult to do. Once parents open their minds up to the possibility that their infant may be suffering from colic, it is actually quite easy to assess. This assessment is initially done through behavioral observation. Parents are usually the ones who make these observations, but it is not uncommon for other family members, friends, neighbors, or child care professionals to observe crying patterns in your baby. The person that spends the most time with him is probably best equipped to track these patterns and report them to you and/or your pediatrician.

If your baby fits Dr. Wessel's "Rule of Threes," then it is likely that he is suffering from some form of colic. In other words, if your baby cries at least three hours per day, three days in a row, for at least three weeks, he will often be given this label by his doctor. Upon hearing this diagnosis, parents are often relieved to know that their baby's relentless crying bouts are not due to a severe medical problem. However, this feeling of relief is quickly replaced with feelings of frustration and helplessness when they learn that there is no cure.

Only under certain circumstances—such as with the diagnosis of infant GERD—can parents rely on the use of medication to relieve their baby's distress. In this case, doctor assessment will be primary in making a formal diagnosis. Although this is a less common cause of colic, it is still prevalent among infants and should be investigated. The following includes specific information about the diagnosis of infant GERD and ways to intervene.

Background

It is interesting how the word *colic* sounds like a terrible disease. Initially, it is not uncommon for parents to deny colic as the problem either due to lack of understanding, fear, or uncertainty. One of the difficulties that most new parents face is trusting their own instincts. This is particularly true for first-time parents. For them, having a newborn at home is a foreign concept. Interestingly, despite this fact, when parents have a colicky infant (whether that baby is their firstborn or their tenth born), they usually know instinctively that something is wrong the moment their baby starts to cry. But when their baby won't stop crying, they may not automatically respond to these cries because of their own uncertainties.

To complicate matters, colic may present itself in different ways, leading to even more confusion for the new parent. As you gain a better understanding of colic, you will begin to see that the way one parent describes a colicky infant will be quite different from the way another parent describes these signs and symptoms. This variation is most often due to the varying causes of the problem, which were outlined in Chapter 1.

Ask Questions

If you are reading this book, you probably already know if your baby is colicky. Most parents are quick to make appointments with their pediatrician upon observing the slightest indication of infant distress. However, if you have any uncertainties in your mind or any additional questions about this diagnosis, I would recommend either an appointment with your pediatrician or a discussion with an advice nurse.

"With knowledge comes power"—I have always liked that quote. Before Tyler was diagnosed with colic, I thought about what the diagnosis of colic would mean. I came to the conclusion that basically he would be fussier, more irritable, and moodier than the average infant. Certainly I could handle that, couldn't I? In order to convince myself, I reminded myself that I was a professional clinical psychologist who had worked with children and teenagers in crisis. For over ten years, I have handled cases that involve physical abuse, sexual assault, eating disorders, self-mutilation, suicide/homicide, substance abuse, and domestic violence. Could a five-day-old infant really be more difficult than that? Only time would tell.

When Tyler began to cry relentlessly for hours at a time in his first week of life, I contacted an advice nurse to get some answers. This was my first course of action. I was afraid, and because it was before business hours, I was contemplating taking him to the emergency room. Most doctor's offices have on-call advice nurses whom you can speak with around the clock. They will contact your pediatrician if they have any questions or need guidance on medical concerns or treatment plans.

After hearing about the night I had experienced with Tyler (when he cried for ten straight hours), the advice nurse informed me that she thought he probably had colic. I had heard the word colic before, but didn't really understand what it was. She explained that many infants suffer from extreme gassiness and become upset, fussy, and cry due to that discomfort shortly after they are born. Due to the fact that Tyler did not exhibit any other distressing symptoms, the nurse told us not to worry and that it was probably just gas. However, she said, we should wait and see if he experienced similar trouble later that evening and if so, to bring him in the following day for a checkup just in case something else was wrong.

I was intrigued by the nurse's response regarding colic during the evening hours. Tyler was doing much better on the early morning that I called. I wondered why there would be a difference between morning and evening gassiness. Therefore, I asked her why she mentioned looking for similar problems in the *evening* but not during the day. She replied that colicky infants often only react during the evening hours. On one hand, I was somewhat relieved to hear that if Tyler did suffer from colic we would at least have a better day than night, but on the other hand, I was not looking forward to the possibility of repeating a night like we already had. Truth be told, it terrified me.

I also talked with the nurse about my concerns for Tyler's lack of sleep and lack of food intake during the long, hard hours the night before. She assured me that although this was not preferable, most babies would not starve themselves and when hungry enough, they will eat. She also stated that when tired enough, they will sleep, and that most likely Tyler would be catching up on his sleep at some point later in the day. The idea of a sleeping baby for several hours was comforting, but the possibility of a non-sleeping baby again at night was highly stressful. After another sleepless night battling the challenges of relentless crying, I was advised by the nurse to bring Tyler in for a checkup to ensure his medical stability. I made an appointment for the next day.

Going to the pediatrician's office with a colicky infant can be a production in and of itself. Let's face it; going anywhere with an inconsolable child is distressing for everyone involved, including those around you. This is even true if the crying is expected in places such as a pediatrician's office. The loud shrill cries that come from a colicky infant are surprisingly intense and rattle even the most experienced person. I remember arriving at our pediatrician's office with Tyler in his usual state of distress. The nurses quickly removed us from the waiting room (which was packed) and put us into a room down the hall in the farthest corner of the building away from all signs of life. Coincidence? Maybe, but Jason, who accompanied me that day, did not think so.

Tyler screamed loudly for twenty minutes straight. We began to worry that we scared all of the doctors and nurses off since nobody had come into our room since we had been escorted down the hall. However, we found some solace in the fact that there would be no way that the medical staff could forget about us because we had a constant screaming reminder for them that we were certain everyone could hear.

One of the doctors in the group opened the door and the first thing that she said was "Wow, your son really has a set of lungs on him. I could hear him all the way down the hallway when I was with another patient." Jason and I smiled for the first time in a long time with a sense of validation. We agreed with her and told her about our situation.

It was hard to communicate with her over Tyler's loud cries. We tried swaying, swinging, singing, etc., during the conversation to try to calm Tyler down, but as usual nothing seemed to work for more than a few minutes.

The doctor did not seem to be bothered by Tyler's screams. However, I was certain she sensed our desperation. Jason and I were grateful to have a medical professional understand and see our struggles. Even more validating, she mentioned that one of her own children had been colicky. Therefore, she was very aware of the struggles we were facing. Although at the time she did not have any definitive answers for us about Tyler, she did state that the diagnosis of colic was likely due to the fact that he was otherwise medically healthy.

Finding answers from your pediatrician and/or advice nurse is the best place to start because of their medical training and expertise. However, another place to find answers or support with colic is in a variety of reading material. Books, magazine articles, and the Internet may all provide you with some information on colic. If you have a colicky infant and find very little time to do anything but soothe your infant, do not be afraid to enlist the help of others. One woman told me she had her mother-in-law read books on parenting while she handled her baby. Another woman stated that her husband collected magazine articles and pamphlets on infant GERD because she did not have the time to do it herself. Upon hearing what the advice nurse had said to me on the phone that day, Jason searched the Internet for information to gain a better understanding of the problem and tips on what we could do about it if indeed Tyler had colic.

Talk with family, friends, and neighbors about your struggles. Do not be afraid to ask them if they had a baby with colic. Remember, one in four babies in America struggle with some form of colic. Interestingly, most families do not talk about these struggles unless they know that you are walking in their shoes. You might be surprised by what you find out and be thankful for the tips that they willingly and enthusiastically offer. At minimum, you may be intrigued to know what has worked for other people in your situation during this very difficult time.

A man once told me that his baby suffered from such a severe case of colic that the only thing that worked was driving their baby in the car. They became so tired from driving in the middle of the night that they had to come up with something else so they could get some sleep. They devised a plan to take down their fence so they could drive their car into their backyard and leave it running next to their open bedroom window (with the exhaust pipe facing away from their window for safety). This way they were able to sleep in their own bed while the baby slept soundly throughout the first half of the night.

My neighbor heard about Tyler's colic and offered some advice about what she did when her son cried relentlessly throughout the day. She told me that she took him for long walks in his stroller. During these walks she wore her earphones and listened to music so that when he did cry, it did not bother her. The exercise made her feel better, got her out of the house, and gave her and her son some relief. Although this was not a cure for his crying bouts, it is a good example of how sometimes finding a coping mechanism can be helpful and get you through a tough time.

Talking with family can also be informative and helpful. I told my mother what the advice nurse and pediatrician said to me regarding the possible diagnosis of colic. My mother knew about colic but had never been around a baby who suffered from it. She said that crying spells with kids in the evening hours were common, which is why many parents of her generation called them the witching hours. Most infants, whether they have colic or not, become fussy during the early evening hours.

This notion intrigues me, particularly since I spend most of my day exploring the human psyche. From both professional and personal experiences, I have been made aware that human beings in general, babies and adults alike, become more irritable around early evening. Think about your own patterns of moods and those of your friends and family members. In doing so you might realize that frequently individuals come home at night feeling tired, hungry, and moodier than usual. Whatever the reason for this shift, it seems to be a more difficult time of day for many people.

My personal belief on this issue is that as individuals age, they are better able to control their various moods. I think that individuals learn how to develop coping mechanisms to soothe themselves so that their moods do not affect them or those around them in highly negative ways. These coping mechanisms may be positive or negative, healthy or unhealthy. In either case, they are adopted by individuals to help alter mood, attitude, or mindset. For example, it is common (maybe too common) for an adult to come home from a long, hard day at work and say, "I could really use a drink" or "Let's relax with some wine tonight." I personally know many adults who feel this way. I also know individuals who go to the gym to exercise in order to wind down from a long day at the office or a hard day with the kids.

Obviously, these are not the only two ways people find to relax. Other individuals might listen to music, cook dinner, read, write, or watch TV. Those who don't sit in front of a computer all day might come home and check email or surf the Net. All of these things seem to help individuals cope with adult witching hours.

Unfortunately, none of these coping mechanisms can be utilized by infants, at least not by themselves. Therefore, I believe that they cry, fuss, and whine instead. This is their way of handling their own feelings of distress. They are communicating to us what they are feeling and that they do not know how to alter these feelings. In time, they will develop coping mechanisms like everyone else, but for now this is all they have, which can be extremely frustrating and difficult for parents.

Interestingly, I believe that parents attempt to engage their infants in some of the coping mechanisms that work for them. How many parents do you know who plop their children down in front of the TV while cooking dinner not only to occupy their interest and keep them out of their way, but also to distract them from the witching hours. Other parents sing to their children, hold them, rock them, and listen to music with them. Whatever the case, parents clearly try to find ways to get through these tougher hours of the day.

For Best Results in Finding Answers

For best results in finding answers to your very important questions, I would recommend several different things. First, make a list of your questions so that when you meet with your pediatrician, advice nurse, or lactation specialist, you cover all of your concerns. It is not uncommon for parents to forget to ask certain questions that seemed incredibly important at the time but have since slipped their minds, only to resurface again at a later time. There is a lot to think about when you have a colicky infant. It is not just the common questions and concerns parents have regarding a newborn, but those that arise when that newborn won't stop crying.

I have heard of numerous stories from parents about the many questions that run through their minds in the midst of the storm of colic. Yet when they get to their doctor's appointment, they suddenly have little to ask because they are in the calm of the storm. However, they remember their burning questions when the storm strikes again (usually after business hours).

These predicaments remind me of having car trouble. Imagine being on the freeway and your engine light goes on. You are not sure if you should pull over to the side of the road, head for the nearest gas station, or take your chances and try to make it to your final destination. You decide to go for it, and luckily you make it to your final destination. During this trip, you are nervous. You are uncertain what will happen along the way and hope for the best. You have no choice but to ignore the clanking noise, squeaking sound, and suspicious smell that filters into your car.

The next day you are forced to miss work, rearrange your schedule, and bring your car in for a checkup. You notice on your way to the mechanic's shop that your engine light has miraculously turned itself off. You assure the technician that it was on the day before. However, despite your assurance, after a quick test ride, he tells you there is absolutely nothing wrong with your car.

Puzzled, you leave for work. On your way to the office you notice the unpredictable light goes on once again. In addition, it is only at this time that you realize you forgot to ask the technician about the sounds and smell that were present while driving yesterday. With these problems reemerging and your car stalling out on the freeway, they are suddenly on the forefront of your mind. With this new information, the technician is better able to assess the problem and find a cause.

When asking questions, give as much detail as possible. Remember, every baby is different. What may be the case for your baby with colic may not be the case for another. In addition, be sure to ask every question you have (thus the importance of making a list). If you have concerns for your baby, no matter how great or small, voice them. Entitle yourself and your baby to information that will calm your fears and potentially diminish your baby's distress.

The most common reason that parents do not ask questions is that they forget them. The second most common reason parents do not ask questions is because they think their questions are insignificant, unimportant, or silly. Remember there is no such thing as a dumb question.

Frequently, it is the questions that do not pertain directly to our infants, but rather to ourselves, that we are reluctant to ask. Concerns pertaining to yourself as a parent are just as significant as those pertaining to your child. For example, I recall a specific concern that I had while I was waiting for my breast milk to come in. Due to the fact that this concern had more to do with me than it did for my baby, I was reluctant to voice it. However, I eventually did address this concern with my OB/GYN and received an incredibly helpful tip.

My concern had to do with breast engorgement. While waiting for my breast milk to come in, my breasts became so engorged that I was in excruciating pain. They were swollen to about the size of footballs, as hard as rocks, black and blue, and so hot that I swear you could have cooked eggs on them. I was told by varying sources not to pump because this could prolong the engorgement phase. Therefore, I struggled with this pain believing I had no other choice.

Breast milk is produced on a supply-and-demand basis. Therefore, the more you stimulate the breast, whether through actual breast-feedings or pumping, the more the body will produce. However, this does not mean that you have to suffer in pain while you wait for your milk to come in. Luckily, I mustered up enough courage to call my doctor and ask what I could do for myself. The receptionist took the call and unfortunately did not have an answer for me. However, she was willing to ask the women in the waiting room for tips on how to decrease this pain.

One woman responded with something that I had never heard before. She recommended that I buy a head of cabbage. She stated that stuffing cabbage leaves into my nursing bras would ease the pain. Ice packs, Tylenol, warm compresses, and hot showers did not work for me, which were also suggested, but cabbage leaves did the trick. They absorbed the heat, decreased the swelling, and relieved the bruising. Who would have thought that a vegetable could provide such a wonderful service to the nursing mother? If I didn't have the courage to ask, I would have never known.

Important Points for Diagnosis

Unlike other infants, the colicky infant rarely stops once the crying begins. Therefore, waiting it out usually does not work. If you have a colicky infant at home, you will probably agree that your baby does not tend to wind down. Instead, you probably have noticed that he can quickly work himself up into a frenzy. It is so common that many parents signify this process with a name. Jason and I called it a "code red." I have also heard names such as "go time," "the meltdown," and "the rising."

Intervening quickly in the midst of this emotional storm is helpful. Therefore, trying the different strategies to soothe your colicky infant outlined in Chapter 5, "Finally an Answer," will be key in finding some relief. Furthermore, knowing the cause will help you decide what intervention strategies to choose. Whatever the cause may be, preparing for the challenges you will face during your baby's relentless crying outbursts is a helpful way to decrease the distress that you and your baby will inevitably experience. Preparation for these challenges will be different for each parent, depending on you and your child's individual needs.

Probably your most important task in preparation will be to investigate your baby's crying pattern. It is extremely helpful to assess the crying pattern that your baby experiences throughout the day and night. Be sure to write this pattern down so that you do not forget it. In your observations, if you are able to establish a consistent pattern of crying, it will undoubtedly be easier for you and your baby to adjust to the storm of colic. If you are not able to track a consistent pattern due to the sporadic nature of your child's colic, then you will face greater difficulties and should prepare for these hurdles. Don't worry, you can overcome these hurdles. I know I did, with practice and patience.

Let's first look at a situation in which a baby has a consistent cry pattern. Let's say your baby cries consistently in the evening hours from 6:00 p.m. until 10:00 p.m. During his crying episode, your focus will most likely be on him. Therefore, there will be little or no time left over to spend with other family members or for yourself. Many families agree that this time of night is often spent as family time. Having a colicky infant present in the home will inevitably disrupt this in some way. I commonly speak with family members who acknowledge their struggles with finding the time to cook dinner, take a shower, clean the house, help their older child with homework, prepare work items, and lay out school clothes for the next day.

These once seemingly simple tasks become difficult and challenging even for the most organized individual. However, knowing that these tasks will be difficult to achieve once 6:00 p.m. comes along allows you to think and plan ahead. Accomplishing as much as possible before the storm hits will allow you to feel less anxious and overwhelmed during those relentless crying hours.

If you are a parent who has a colicky infant with no set pattern of crying, your job may be more difficult, but again not impossible. Tyler was one of these cases, and although it was difficult, I was able to devise a plan that worked for me to preserve sanity in my household. The biggest lesson that I learned through my own experience was to take advantage of every single moment that he was not crying. For example, I learned to sleep when he slept, take showers when he was calm, and prepare easy meals that could be made in five minutes. You can find these meals at most large grocery stores. They are often displayed in a separate section that is specifically designated for the working mother.

This type of planning allows you to feel more prepared for the relentless crying spurts that you will encounter throughout the day.

Whether your baby has a consistent pattern of crying or a sporadic one, your preparation should include a plan for both emotional and behavioral relief.

Remember that the crying spurts that take place in the evening hours are usually most difficult for parents. As discussed earlier, most human beings experience the witching hours. During this time of day you may be used to taking care of yourself and not having to be responsible for someone else. This adjustment is difficult for parents whose infants don't have colic. It is even more difficult for parents with colicky infants.

Preparation for bedtime can be particularly challenging. Colicky infants do not generally cry themselves to sleep, not even during bedtime hours. Instead, they continue to cry relentlessly (sometimes for hours) causing them increased distress and wakefulness. Constant crying at any time of day takes a toll on your emotions, however, this is particularly true when you are tired and would like to get to bed yourself. The fact that a colicky infant's cry is often described as bone-chilling, high-pitched, and screeching makes this even more difficult to bear.

Postpartum Depression

When a person struggles with a particular issue or is in the midst of a challenging situation, he or she is often at higher risk for problems such as depression or anxiety. In these situations, diagnosing the problem of colic is not the only diagnosis that may need to be made. Recognizing the signs and symptoms of postpartum depression in the mother may also be a necessity. As you will see below, it is common for women to experience some form of postpartum depression due to a mix of biological, social, and psychological factors.

There are different severity levels of postpartum depression. The mildest level is called "postpartum blues" or "baby blues." Symptoms include mood instability, sadness, weepiness, and anxiety. Approximately 80 percent of women experience these symptoms, which usually start one week after delivery and last for three to six weeks. The most common causes of these blues are: (1) rapid hormonal changes in the body, (2) emotional and physical stress of labor and delivery, including physical discomforts, (3) disappointments (i.e., C-section versus vaginal birth, breast-feeding difficulties, lack of spousal support, etc.), and (4) sleep deprivation.

True postpartum depression is more severe than postpartum blues. It is experienced by approximately 15 to 20 percent of mothers. Symptoms include feeling overwhelmed and/or hopeless, sad and/or irritable; exhibiting poor concentration and indecisiveness; and having sleeping and/or eating problems. A loss of interest or pleasure in activities that the woman used to find interesting or pleasurable, decreased libido, and a lowered frustration tolerance may also be apparent. In addition, these women often feel a lack of connectedness toward their newborns.

Risk factors for the development of this disorder include having had a previous postpartum depression (50 to 80 percent more likely), depression or anxiety during pregnancy, family history of depression or anxiety, social isolation, and an inadequate support system. In addition, there is some research that indicates that a history of premenstrual syndrome (PMS) or premenstrual dysphoric disorder (PMDD) can increase a woman's risk of developing postpartum depression. It is important to note that a thyroid dysfunction can mimic signs of postpartum depression and thus should be ruled out by a medical doctor.

The most severe level of postpartum depression is postpartum psychosis. It is uncommonly seen, affecting approximately 1 in 1,000 women. However, it is extremely dangerous and should be treated immediately due to its lethality rate. This disorder has a 5 percent suicide rate and 4 percent infanticide rate. It usually appears within the first postpartum week.

Symptoms for postpartum psychosis include visual or auditory hallucinations (seeing or hearing things that are not really there), delusional thinking (strongly held irrational or illogical beliefs such as denial of baby's birth or need to kill their baby), and delirium (disturbance of consciousness or a change in cognition) and/or mania (abnormally and persistently elevated, expansive, or irritable mood). Risk factors for the development of this disorder are a previous postpartum psychotic or bipolar episode and a personal or family history of psychosis, bipolar disorder, or schizophrenia.

All three levels of postpartum depression are treatable. It is important for women to reach out and utilize the support systems around them so that they are not isolated. Isolation can worsen depressive symptoms. Depression can be an incredibly debilitating disorder. Two wonderful resources for women struggling with feelings of postpartum depression—regardless of the level of severity—are: (1) Postpartum Support International: (805) 967-7636 or www.postpartum.net and (2) Depression after Delivery: (800) 944-4773 or www.depressionafterdelivery.com. In addition, women can contact their local hospitals, doctors, and pediatricians who usually have a wealth of resources on support groups and nearby therapists who specialize in the treatment of postpartum depression.

When I was pregnant, I remember reading in a parenting magazine that women who are most susceptible to postpartum depression fit the following three criteria: (1) career women who work full time, (2) women who like to keep busy, and (3) women who do not have support. At the time, I found it interesting and a bit scary that I fit all three criteria. I have worked full time since the age of twenty-three. I definitely am a person who likes to stay busy and I did not have any family living in the area to provide consistent support with motherhood. I wondered if I would struggle with any type of postpartum depression.

As mentioned above, one of the risk factors for postpartum depression is the presence of a family history of depression, more specifically, postpartum depression. My mother never experienced postpartum depression, but my aunt did. Recognizing that I was at risk, I was determined to avoid the development of this disorder. It is important to note that depression is not always avoidable. In fact, it is often a biological process that is out of the individual's control. However, being in the mental health profession, I knew exactly what I could do to lower my chances of developing postpartum blues or a full depression.

Depression can be caused due to biological factors (i.e., chemical imbalances in the brain or hormonal fluctuations), situational factors, or a combination of the two. If caused by biological factors, most psychiatrists will prescribe the use of medication, particularly if this depression is severe. Research clearly shows that if a depression is left untreated, the individual is at greater risk for a recurrence of depression that is more intense and episodes that are closer together in time. For example, a woman who is diagnosed with depression in her teenage years may remit from the problem without any treatment after only a few weeks. However, that same woman will be at much higher risk to have another depressive episode later in life, which will be more severe and longer lasting. In addition, if left untreated once again, the next episode is more likely to arise in a shorter time span than that between the first and second episodes and with much more significant signs and symptoms.

Depression caused by situational factors can often be treated without the use of medication. Situational factors such as a life phase change (e.g., having a baby) can cause even the most stable individual to feel anxious and/or depressed. Many people have trouble understanding this fact. They imagine new parents being excited and elated, not depressed. I know I imagined what it would be like to have a precious newborn in my life and envisioned myself rejoicing in my baby's presence. However, with feelings of excitement also come feelings of uncertainty and fear. This is particularly true for parents with a colicky infant.

Most new parents do not think about the unexpected turns that will be ever present in their lives once their baby is born. Instead, they think about meeting their baby for the first time and reveling in the simple joys of parenthood. Unfortunately, when faced with the problem of colic, many parents begin to think the unspeakable. For example, it is common for parents to ask themselves, "Did we make a terrible mistake?" or "Should we give our baby up for adoption?" In addition, thoughts such as "I don't know what I am doing" or "I am not cut out to be a mother" are common. These thoughts often turn into strongly held beliefs such as "I am a terrible parent" or "I can't do this anymore."

These questions, thoughts, and beliefs are usually not shared with others for fear that the parent will be judged, criticized, misunderstood, or punished in some way. Many parents will not even share these thoughts with their significant others. I know I personally struggled with this dilemma. My husband is my best friend and my soul mate. I remember thinking that if I could not open up to him I could not open up to anyone, and there were many times I could not open up to him.

My experience with motherhood, at least initially, was the complete opposite of my experience at work. I have always enjoyed my work. It has a purpose and makes me feel important. At work, I feel that I am making a difference in the world. Mothering a colicky infant was not like this for me. There were many times that I felt completely useless! I often believed that I couldn't make a single bit of difference in the life of my own child. As I am sure you can imagine, that is a terrible feeling to have. I often wondered at the time if a mother without a colicky infant could fully understand this feeling. I know now that with varying circumstances these feelings come up for a variety of parents during different stages of parenting. I have worked with many parents professionally who have expressed similar thoughts and feelings.

One particular situation clearly exemplifies the increasing negative feelings I had about myself and motherhood and the realization that I was slipping into a depression. Tyler was only seven days old when Jason and I were driving late at night in an attempt to soothe him. Since Tyler's birth, due to my C-section I was not yet permitted to drive. I had been cooped up in a hospital bed or stuck in our house for a full week and it was starting to get to me. I have always been a person who needs exercise and activity to feel psychologically and physically healthy. However, as most of you know, this is next to impossible with a colicky newborn at home.

Feeling locked up with nowhere to go, I was beginning to show some signs of the postpartum blues. At first, I was not particularly alarmed by these symptoms, but I also recognized that they could worsen quickly and easily. I decided to share my concerns with Jason that night. It was difficult to talk over the loud cries of our colicky baby, but we managed to have some sort of intelligible conversation.

I began to think about what I needed to do in order to stop the depression from worsening. I created an action plan for myself. First, I knew I needed to keep active. Exercise, no matter how much, is always helpful both biologically and emotionally. The most effective treatment for depression is a combination of antidepressant drugs and psychotherapy; however, recent research suggests that regular exercise may also be an effective way to improve a person's mood. A study conducted at Duke University's Medical Center compared the effects of exercise and drug therapy in treating depression in older people. Results indicated that participants who used a combination of exercise and drug therapy improved the fastest. In fact, following this treatment, approximately 68 percent of them were no longer classified as clinically depressed.

Second, I knew that forming some sort of daily routine would be useful. It would give my day purpose. I needed to feel that my life had a purpose. Of course, pushing myself to follow a daily routine when I was depressed was a challenge. Lack of motivation is one of the key characteristics of depression. However, logically I knew it would be well worth the effort. One way to improve motivation and the chances of sticking to a daily routine is to enlist the help of others. A friend or family member that is willing to check in with you and support your efforts is often highly helpful. One woman told me that when she was in the midst of a postpartum depression, her mother called her every morning to make sure she was out of bed. Another told me that her neighbor, who had also suffered from a postpartum depression, came over every morning with a cup of coffee to help her start her day.

I was developing a lot of negative and self-defeating thoughts very early on about my ability to parent. I knew this needed to stop because it can lead to an increase in depressive symptoms. Therefore, my third objective would include fighting against and challenging these unproductive thoughts. In fact, this objective would need to be at the top of my priority list. Thinking positively (no matter how Pollyannaish this may seem) helps to eliminate negative thinking. Interestingly, enjoyable exercise can also help accomplish this goal. It can distract a person long enough to break the vicious cycle of pessimistic thinking.

Last but not least, I knew I would need to utilize the support systems around me. Unfortunately, all of our family members were living out of state, but I knew there had to be plenty of resources out there for new mothers. It would just be a matter of finding them. If Tyler continued with his colicky bouts, I would need all the support I could get. I actually started thinking about hiring a nanny to help me out and give me some relief. I was sure I could find someone who would be willing to work at night if necessary.

It is difficult for many parents to find professional child care. This task is even harder for parents with a colicky infant. Every parent desires a safe and dependable provider who would not purposely or even accidentally cause harm or detriment to their child. These child care providers are often difficult to find. Having a colicky infant can complicate this search.

Many parents have been at their wits' end when their baby won't stop crying. Although they are certain that they would never harm their child, they can understand how it happens. Shaking a child, yelling at him, leaving him alone in a room unsupervised, even throwing him out a window have all been done by parents all over the world in an attempt to find some relief from the constant crying. Therefore, parents worry that even the most seasoned, dependable, patient, and loving care provider could "lose it" when their baby won't stop crying for hours.

If you are looking for dependable child care for your colicky infant, you will find that there are many places to search. Due to the added challenges that a colicky infant brings to the world of child care, I would caution you against hiring someone who is not very well trained and/or inexperienced with infants. Preferably, you would want someone who is clearly experienced and able to handle a crying infant for hours at a time. However, this is not often easy to find and in many cases it is difficult to assess until the provider is on the job. Therefore, I would highly encourage you to spend as much time with your potential child care provider as possible before leaving your baby alone with her. This will give you the opportunity to observe her abilities and interactions with your child and decrease any fears that you might have. Only you can ultimately decide what is right for your baby. Take the time to check references, check credentials, check police lists, and observe; it will be well worth it in the end for your infant's well-being and your peace of mind.

CHAPTER REVIEW

Ask Questions
* Make a doctor's appointment.
* Call the advice nurse.
* Speak with a lactation specialist.
* Gain information through reading.
* Talk to other parents.

For Best Results in Finding Answers
* Make a list of your questions so that you cover all concerns.
* Ask every question you have. There are no dumb questions.
* When asking questions, give as much detail as possible to those with whom you are speaking.
* Remember every baby is different. What may be the case for one may not be the case for another.
* Tip for breast-feeding: Place a few drops of formula on your nipple from a bottle to entice your newborn to latch on.

The Colic Diagnosis
* Colicky babies do not generally cry themselves to sleep but instead continue to cry relentlessly (sometimes for hours).
* Colicky infants do not tend to wind down; instead they tend to wind up and work themselves into a frenzy.
* Colicky infants do not always follow a pattern. What calms them at a given moment may excite them at another.
* Unlike other infants, when crying begins the colicky infant will rarely stop crying on his own, so waiting it out usually does not work. Instead, intervening quickly is helpful.

* Unlike other babies, cries from a colicky infant can be described as bone-chilling, high-pitched, and screeching.
* It is not uncommon for parents to rush their colicky infant to the emergency room in fear that he is in horrific pain.

Important Information for Mothers

* Breast-feeding mothers may have to wait for up to seven days after giving birth for their milk to come in.
* Engorged breasts can be soothed with ice packs (a bag of frozen peas works best), cabbage leaves (to stuff, not to eat), warm compresses, hot showers, and Tylenol (consult with your doctor before using).
* Most babies will not starve themselves; when hungry enough, they will eat.
* Sleep deprivation has its own set of consequences.
* Postpartum depression is common. Be sure to look for signs and symptoms and intervene immediately.

Postpartum Depression

Risk Factors

* There are a variety of different factors that place women at risk.
* Some women are more susceptible than others.

Severity Levels

* Eighty percent of women experience the mildest level, which is called "postpartum blues" or "baby blues."
* Approximately 15 percent of mothers experience true postpartum depression, which is more severe than postpartum blues.

* The most severe level of postpartum depression is postpartum psychosis. Although this is uncommonly seen, affecting only an estimated 1 in 1,000 women, it is extremely dangerous and should be treated immediately due to its lethality rate (with a 5 percent suicide rate and 4 percent infanticide rate).
* All three levels of postpartum depression are treatable.

Intervention

* Seek support in the form of individual therapy, group therapy, telephone help lines, and/or reading materials.
* Keep active.
* Set a daily routine.
* Fight against and challenge unproductive thoughts in order to eliminate negative thinking.
* Utilize the support systems around you, however big or small they may be.

Chapter 4

Treatment Approaches for Specific Causes

Finding relief from the distressing situation of colic will be similar to your journey to diagnose the problem. In other words, it is important to consult with your pediatrician, advice nurse, lactation specialist, or counselor to find answers to your questions as well as to obtain information on specific strategies.

Pediatrician

Since the most common theory indicates that colic is caused by some sort of trouble with the digestive system, Jason and I decided to consult our pediatrician first to ask what could be done in order to test this theory. I highly recommend that all parents do the same. Make an in-office appointment so your pediatrician can get a flavor of exactly what you are talking about. Set the appointment for the time when your baby is normally colicky. Although this is often much more stressful on the parent, it allows the doctor to directly observe the problem.

Many parents of colicky infants worry that others—including their pediatrician—might think they are exaggerating how bad the crying really is. Presenting the problem directly will decrease these worries and provide you with a thorough medical assessment.

Initial Strategies

Our pediatrician gave us a list of calming techniques to try with Tyler. There are several initial strategies that you probably have already been using. If they are working, stick with them. Any strategy that works to provide both you and your baby with some relief is a good one for your family as long as it is safe and not detrimental to any family member. When Jason and I first encountered Tyler's nonstop crying, we had no idea what to do. Instinctively, we both held him and rocked him. My mother had some luck with a pacifier and singing a German lullaby in his ear. Unfortunately for us, none of these interventions worked for long periods of time. Just as Tyler seemed to be soothed with one strategy, he would start crying again. This is not uncommon.

Many parents admit that their infant does well temporarily with one technique but then does not seem to like it the next time it is used. The reason behind some of this may be that the technique in the given moment provides your baby with a distraction. A change in his environment may intrigue him and cause him to stop crying as it catches his attention. However, once he is accustomed to the change in his environment, he may find his way back into the recent state of affairs.

When I first tried to soothe Tyler, I tried all the strategies. I swaddled Tyler tight in his blanket, rocked him, sang to him, and even danced with him. When none of this worked as successfully as I would have liked, I tried to change his environment. I remember one evening after four hours of nonstop crying; I wrapped Tyler up in his blanket and walked outside of my house. I needed some air and thought the cool spring night might help Tyler as well. Surprisingly, it did. I don't know if it was the change in scenery, the change in temperature, or something else, but his cries became less intense.

Below is a list of initial strategies that were offered to us by our pediatrician. Since they are all highly published strategies, many of them are attempted by most parents before they request a specific appointment with their pediatrician to assess for colic. If you are unsure about the use of any of these techniques, contact your pediatrician and consult him or her on varying strategies to accomplish the goal of infant relief.

Vibration

This highly publicized technique can be utilized in several different ways. The key to this strategy is to find a way to cause some sort of soft vibration for your baby. A drive in the car or a rest on the dryer can accomplish this task. If you choose to utilize the former technique, note that stop-and-go driving due to traffic lights is not as helpful. In fact, it often causes the baby to wake up and develop greater fatigue and distress. In contrast, freeway driving (at least in most cases) works better to calm the baby down. This provides him with a continuous vibration. If you choose to utilize the latter technique, put your baby in a safe apparatus (e.g., car seat or bassinet) and then place him on top of the dryer. Then turn the dryer on.

Note: For safety reasons *always* strap your baby into the chosen apparatus when possible, *never* leave him unattended, and *never* mistakenly put him into the dryer.

White Noise

Many things can produce white noise. For example, a vacuum cleaner, a static TV or radio station, a blender, and even a sound machine can produce this noise. Perhaps the most common way to produce this noise is to shush in the baby's ear. White noise mimics the sound of blood flow in utero and thus makes infants feel right at home.

Bathing

This technique often helps to soothe a colicky infant. However, it often takes some practice by parents and some getting used to by infants. In fact, this new experience for infants may not be enjoyable until after several attempts. If you choose to utilize this strategy, place your baby in a bathtub, making sure that the water is lukewarm or at room temperature. Use baby soap or shampoo that is proven safe for infants less than six months of age.

Massage Therapy

Infants can often be soothed with infant massage. Training in these specific techniques so not to harm your baby is imperative. Ask your pediatrician for information on training opportunities. In general, clockwise circles starting at the top of the baby's limbs and working your way downward is indicated by these massage specialists. Infant massage can be performed on every limb as well as on the torso. Too much pressure can be harmful to your infant. Avoid the head area.

Note: Use powder or cream that is proven safe for infants less than six months of age to massage more easily.

Outcome

As mentioned above, it is possible that either all or some of the above techniques will only provide your baby with some temporary distraction and not lead to long-term relief. If this is the case, do not hesitate to speak with your pediatrician once again to obtain more answers. For example, one of the specific reasons that your baby won't stop crying might be the fact that he is suffering from infant GERD. Therefore, it is important for your pediatrician to assess for this and either diagnose it or rule it out. Another specific reason that your baby won't stop crying may be the fact that he is suffering from food allergies. This also should be assessed. These two specific causes are discussed in greater detail following. The good news is that there are proven treatment approaches for both of these specific causes.

Specific Causes

Infant GERD or Gassiness

It is always important to investigate the various medical reasons for colic. If your pediatrician diagnoses your infant with colic, he should immediately investigate the possible causes. Remember, the two most common medical reasons for colic are: (1) gassiness, or (2) infant gastroesophageal reflux disease (GERD). In order for these to be properly diagnosed, your pediatrician will need information about your baby's crying patterns. Therefore, be prepared to give him a detailed description of when your baby cries and for how long. This important information is particularly helpful to your doctor when investigating the possibility of infant GERD.

If an individual suffers from GERD, it means that acid and other stomach contents repeatedly flow back up into the esophagus. A valve called the *lower esophageal sphincter* (LES) opens during normal digestion to allow food to pass into the stomach. It then closes once the food is inside the stomach so that food and stomach acid cannot escape. If the LES is weak or if it does not work at the right time, then both will escape and flow back up into the esophagus. If this happens repetitively, your child probably has GERD.

Interestingly, every child experiences some form of acid reflux at some time. This is also true for adults. Therefore, it is the repetitive nature of the problem that doctors look for to warrant this diagnosis in infancy and childhood. The most common symptoms of infant GERD are: (1) frequent or recurrent vomiting, (2) frequent or persistent cough, and (3) heartburn, gas, or abdominal pain. By the time the infant is twelve to twenty-four months old; some additional symptoms can be noted, such as losing weight, growing more slowly than expected, refusing to eat, and having a scratchy or hoarse voice.

Many babies frequently spit up. This should not be confused with frequent or recurrent vomiting. Parents often are able to tell the difference. However, if you are unsure, consult your pediatrician. Reports given to the pediatrician by parents through the use of their own observations are usually sufficient for the doctor to make a diagnosis of infant GERD. However, under certain circumstances the doctor may request additional tests to ascertain the problem. Tests commonly recommended by pediatricians are: (1) the pH probe, (2) the barium swallow or upper GI series, (3) the upper GI endoscopy, and (4) a gastric emptying study. As you will see, most of these tests are designed for older children and adults.

The pH probe is the best test to diagnose acid reflux; however, physicians do note that it does not always recognize the condition. For this test, the patient is instructed to swallow a long, thin tube which has a probe located on the tip. The tip measures levels of stomach acids at the lower part of the esophagus.

The Barium swallow or upper GI series is a special X-ray test that uses barium to highlight the esophagus, stomach, and upper part of the small intestines. These highlighted areas help the doctor to identify problems more effectively in these areas. In particular, physicians look for abnormalities such as obstructions or narrowing.

The upper GI endoscopy is a test that uses an instrument called an endoscope. An endoscope is a thin, flexible tube that has a light on it. This tube allows the doctor to look directly inside the esophagus, stomach, and upper part of the small intestine to identify any problem areas.

Gastric emptying is a test that uses a special camera to identify problem areas and assess the cause of acid reflux. In order to perform the test, the individual is required to drink milk or eat food that is mixed with a radioactive chemical. The chemical is followed through the gastrointestinal tract using the special camera.

Although infant GERD is not difficult to diagnose, it is often left undiagnosed. This is due to a variety of reasons. First, parents are often completely unaware that infants have the potential to suffer from acid reflux. Since babies are unable to verbally communicate their distress to others, parents are not privileged with the details of their experience. Second, babies often outgrow this problem. As mentioned numerous times before, parents are told by several sources that the only thing they can do for a colicky infant is wait it out. If this is what they do, then the crying eventually will cease when the problem is outgrown. Third, spitting up is commonly confused with recurring vomiting. Since spitting up is common among infants and nothing to be concerned about, parents do not report the problem to their pediatrician. Lastly, parents do not realize that there is a cure for infant GERD. If this is the reason for your infant's colic, then you will be happy to know that there is a very specific and often highly successful treatment plan.

Remember that in order to have a successful treatment plan, it is first important to understand what causes the problem. This is no different in the case of infant GERD. What causes acid reflux in infants is different than what causes acid reflux in children and adults. Most of the time, acid reflux in infants is due to the lack of coordination of the gastrointestinal tract. Remember, infants have an immature digestive system, which is not fully developed until they are approximately one hundred days old. For infants who are otherwise healthy, this problem occurs until their system matures.

In older children and adults there are many possible causes of GERD. In general, anything that causes the LES to relax or anything that increases the pressure below the LES can cause acid reflux and lead to GERD. More specifically, things such as being overweight, eating right before bed, overeating, and eating certain foods or beverages can cause acid reflux. In addition, more recent research indicates that secondhand smoke and certain medications can lead to this problem in children and adults.

The good news is that there are treatment interventions for infant GERD. Most doctors recommend that elevating the head of the baby's crib, bassinet, or basket can reduce the chances of acid reflux and at the same time will not harm the baby. Placing the baby into an upright position both during and after feedings for approximately thirty minutes is also often helpful in reducing the chances of acid reflux. This intervention can be used as a preventative measure and also poses no risk of harm for the infant. In addition, doctors under their supervision may recommend thickening bottle-feedings with cereal, along with changing feeding schedules, trying solid foods, and avoiding foods that are highly acidic.

If infant GERD is severe or does not get better with time, your doctor may recommend the use of medication as a treatment intervention. Over-the-counter medications primarily help with the problem of abdominal pain due to gassiness. For example, Mylicon drops, gripe water, and Babies Tum-Ease are all examples of what your doctor, lactation specialist, or advice nurse may recommend.

Mylicon drops are an FDA-approved product. Most pediatricians feel comfortable recommending this product for infant use. However, some do not under special circumstances, so it is always important to consult with your pediatrician first. Mylicon drops are simply used to help expel gas. They are similar to Gas-X for adults. Like any other product, be prepared for the possibility that this product may not help. However, if you notice that your baby is suffering from gassiness that is causing him distress, it is an option to try.

Gripe water is a product that originally came from England and is now being manufactured in the United States. It is often given to babies who are colicky in order to soothe their stomachs. It contains two simple ingredients: ginger and fennel. Ginger and fennel have been shown to be beneficial for easing nausea and pain due to stomach upset, even in adults. This product contains no fillers, binders, artificial flavors, artificial color, yeast, wheat, gluten, soy, dairy, or starch. Therefore, some professionals will recommend it over some of the other products that are manufactured for the same purposes, such as Babies Tum-Ease.

Babies Tum-Ease is a product that is sold at many organic grocery stores. Like gripe water, it contains ginger and fennel, but also contains dill, kosher vegetable glycerin, and sodium bicarbonate in a base of filtered water. The label on the product indicates that these botanicals are carefully harvested to their optimal potency and that they are either cultivated without the use of chemicals, preservatives, herbicides, pesticides, fumigation, and irradiation or harvested wild in their natural habitat.

Tyler often seemed to struggle with gassiness and stomach discomfort. There were times we could actually hear him digesting his food and could tell that it was distressing for him. If your infant is experiencing discomfort due to his immature digestive system, then a product like gripe water might provide him with some relief. Giving this product to your baby either directly before a feeding or directly after a feeding has proven to be most successful. Since every baby is different, you will need to determine through trial and error which way will be most helpful for your child.

For example, the first time I gave Tyler some gripe water was before an evening feeding. Unfortunately, after this feeding he still seemed to be uncomfortable. The next morning I decided to give him the gripe water *after* his feeding. This seemed to work much better for him. I could actually hear the gripe water working. It sounded as if his stomach was gurgling. I could immediately tell it was helping him digest his food. In addition, he liked the taste of it, which made it easy to administer. Gripe water can be purchased at most birthing hospitals. It can also be purchased online at a variety of baby stores and baby websites, such as babybliss.com.

Unlike the medicines listed above, there are medications that can only be prescribed by a doctor for your infant in the case of infant GERD. These medications are recommended for a variety of reasons. For example, a doctor may prescribe a medication that will improve intestinal coordination or one that will neutralize or decrease stomach acid. In either case, medications have potential side effects. Therefore, it is important to discuss any potential side effects with your pediatrician. For example, Reglan is proven to be effective in treating intestinal coordination, but has the potential for serious side effects.

Conversely, medications that neutralize or decrease stomach acid for the most part are safe. However, at high doses they too can cause some side effects such as diarrhea or sleepiness. These medications include either antacids such as Mylanta or Maalox or acid blockers such as Nexium, Prevacid, or Zantac.

Researchers are uncertain if decreasing stomach acid in infants lessens acid reflux. However, many parents attest to the fact that these types of medications changed their lives within a matter of hours. One woman stated, "My baby cried for hours following each feeding for over one month. On medicine she was a completely different baby. She barely cried at all."

Another possible treatment intervention is surgery. Surgery is not usually needed to treat GERD in children. However, when it is necessary a procedure called the *nissen fundoplication* is most commonly performed. During the procedure, the top part of the stomach is wrapped around the esophagus to create a cuff that can potentially prevent the occurrence of acid reflux. Even though the procedure is often effective, it is usually the last strategy utilized due to the risk involved. Therefore, once again it is important to discuss the potential risks as well as the potential benefits with your pediatrician before deciding to utilize surgery as a treatment plan.

In addition, there are side effects to this procedure. For example, nissen fundoplication causes gagging and retching. In extreme forms, both of these can actually undo the surgical procedure. One woman I met in a support group once talked about her son's experience with this procedure. She stated, "Our son's surgery came completely undone following some intense gagging."

If your doctor determines that your baby suffers from colic due to infant GERD, there are medical treatments that can be employed to correct the problem.

Therefore, it is worthwhile speaking with your pediatrician about the signs and symptoms that your infant exhibits during feeding times. For more detailed information on infant GERD, visit the website: infantrefluxdisease.com. This website provides a wealth of information regarding diagnosis, causes, and treatments.

Lactation Specialist

A lactation specialist is another person that you can consult with to investigate possible causes of colic and learn about specific treatment approaches. This is often the last person that parents think to consult, particularly if breast-feeding is going well for mother and child. Many parents have never even heard of a lactation specialist and have no idea what their area of expertise encompasses. It is common that the first and only time parents are introduced to a lactation specialist and learn about their area of expertise is in the hospital after delivery.

Most hospitals routinely offer a free consultation with this expert before discharging mother and infant as a way to assure that questions regarding breast or bottle-feedings are answered properly. Lactation specialists provide several services. They are highly knowledgeable about all lactation issues as well as lactation paraphernalia (e.g., nursing bras, breast pumps, milk storage units, etc.).

When Tyler's pediatrician diagnosed him with colic after ruling out possible medical causes, she recommended a consultation with a lactation specialist. She stated that a problem with breast-feeding sometimes causes colic. For example, if a baby does not latch onto the breast correctly or if a mother has a low milk supply, then the baby might cry because he is hungry. In most cases, mothers are unaware of this problem, particularly if they are able to breast-feed their baby. In other words, they assume their baby is getting what he needs simply because he is sucking ferociously on the breast.

It is important for mothers to remember that a recommendation to see a lactation specialist is a positive thing and should not be viewed as a failure. I bring this up for good reason. I frequently heard mothers blame themselves for the difficulties they had with breast-feeding. Breast-feeding is a new skill for both mother and infant. It must be learned. Although babies know how to suck instinctively, they are not familiar with a nipple until it is put in front of them. Blaming yourself for breast-feeding challenges does not serve a positive purpose and doing so will inevitably lead to increased frustration and sadness.

One woman I met in a breast-feeding support group told me that she broke down in tears when her doctor recommended she see a lactation specialist. He was convinced that she had a low milk supply and that her baby was hungry. She cringed at the thought of not breast-feeding properly as the thought "I am starving my baby" echoed through her head. The thought that she could be the cause of her baby's distress was awful for her. Another woman in the group shared a similar experience. When she found out that she was not breast-feeding correctly, her initial response was to scream. The possibility fed right into her insecurities about being an inept mother, something she believed nobody else in the world could understand.

Most men are not disturbed by this possibility in the slightest. I know Jason was not. I believe this lack of disturbance is not because men do not care, but rather because with this particular situation, they do not experience feelings of self-blame. After all, they are not the ones breast-feeding the baby or the ones with a possible deficiency. In our case, Jason wanted an action plan. We were running out of ideas and needed answers.

I made an appointment with a lactation specialist right away. Most lactation specialists have offices located at the birthing hospital. Jason took time off work and accompanied me to the appointment. Our specialist's name was Pat. She was the most competent, soothing individual I have ever met. You could tell she felt incredibly comfortable with infants. She gracefully picked Tyler up and held him with ease despite his relentless cries. It was as if she did not even hear him screaming in her ear. Pat commented on Tyler's beauty and size and never said a word about his crying. From our conversation on the phone, she knew why we were there and had expected his colicky outbursts.

What to Expect

Most consultation sessions will involve an evaluation of the mother breast-feeding her baby through behavioral observation. Therefore, scheduling the appointment during a probable feeding hour is preferable. This way the specialist can easily observe the breast-feeding process to assess and comment on it during the designated period. Initially, I was uncomfortable having someone critique my breast-feeding methods. Many women feel anxious during this type of evaluation. In an extreme case, a woman may even exhibit signs and symptoms of performance anxiety, such as sweating, dizziness, nausea, and fainting. If you are susceptible to this type of anxiety, remember that the breast-feeding evaluation has been set up to help you, not to harm you, so there is nothing to fear. The specialist's task is to teach, guide, and support you, not to judge, criticize, or blame you.

Before the evaluation begins, the lactation specialist will weigh the baby. This is done to establish a baseline weight, which will be compared to the baby's weight following the feeding session. Some lactation specialists weigh babies three times during a consultation. They will obtain the baseline weight first, and then a weight after each breast is drained of its milk. This comparison yields an estimate of how much milk is produced in each breast.

Be prepared for a physical evaluation of the breast before and after feedings. A lactation specialist may request to feel your breast to see if it is full of milk before you begin the feeding and empty once the feeding is complete. It is usually easier for a woman to tell when her breast is full of milk than when it is totally empty. When the breast is full, it is physically larger by sight, heavier than normal, and tender to the touch. It is more difficult to tell when the breast is totally empty. Many women feed their babies for a designated amount of time, during which they see their breast become smaller, feel it lessen in weight, and notice a decrease in tenderness through touch. However, an initial change in these three factors does not necessarily indicate that the breast is totally empty. Pat noted that the breast will feel soft and look deflated when the milk is gone.

During the evaluation, your lactation specialist will most likely engage you in conversation and ask direct questions about breast-feeding positions, technique, and schedules. For example, Pat asked me if I was physically comfortable while breast-feeding. She noted that being physically relaxed was important and leads to greater success and positive feelings toward the breast-feeding experience. She showed me different positions in which to hold the baby while breast-feeding that proved to be more relaxing and comfortable for both me and Tyler. The football hold was one of my favorites when Tyler was little. This hold is exactly what it sounds like—you hold your baby face up under your arm like a football.

Pat also commented on my breast-feeding technique. During the evaluation she observed that Tyler's mouth did not open as wide as it could have around my nipple. She asked if I was getting sore nipples from breast-feeding. I told her that I was and she showed me how to help Tyler latch on to more of the breast in order to avoid nipple tenderness. She instructed me to rub my nipple or finger against his cheek or under his chin. As I practiced these techniques, he naturally turned toward my nipple and latched onto my breast more securely. This is called the *rooting reflex*. Tyler opened his mouth wider than I had ever seen before and instinctively started sucking.

Pat asked questions about the length of time that Tyler usually fed. I explained that it varied because he often fell asleep on the breast. She showed me what I could do to keep him awake during his feedings at least until he was full. She tickled his feet, touched his face, and looked directly into his eyes as she engaged him with her words. Tyler stared right back at her as if he could understand everything she was saying. She noted that he might not be getting enough to eat and therefore was waking up sooner than usual.

Take advantage of your time with your lactation specialist. Share your concerns and discuss possible solutions. Parents often have a variety of feeding concerns. This is particularly true for mothers who are breast-feeding. For example, one concern I had with Tyler was that if he fell asleep on the breast, I could not take him off without his awakening. For most babies, this temporary awakening would not be a problem. However, for a colicky infant it is often a huge problem because once the baby wakes up, he cannot easily fall back asleep, which inevitably leads to a new cycle of screaming. This was particularly true for Tyler. Taking him off the breast almost always led to endless hours of crying.

To prevent this from happening, I decided early on not to move him if he was sleeping on my breast. It got to the point where I was scared to even try. Sometimes he would stay in my lap for two hours before waking up from his nap. My arm would fall asleep, my back would hurt, and I would get a cramp in my leg, but I would not dare move because the alternative was worse.

Pat commented that, although understandable, letting Tyler sleep on me for hours after breast-feeding did not give me the opportunity for any type of rest or personal time. Most parents use the time when their baby is napping to accomplish tasks at home, address personal needs, and interact with others. It is a break that all new parents need and deserve, even more so when they have a colicky infant.

In my case, I felt so relieved when Tyler was sleeping because he was peaceful and quiet that I never thought about it as a loss. In fact, it was one of the moments that I actually enjoyed my baby the most. I could watch him lovingly and enjoy his company. I was not sure if I was willing to give up this routine—particularly because I knew there would be a large emotional and physical price to pay if I chose to do so. In my mind, it wasn't really even an option unless we could find some way to stop the colicky screaming. Pat had a few suggestions for us. She asked us to try transferring his mouth from the breast to a finger or to a pacifier. She explained that this would not feel like a loss for him, but rather like a transition. This trick worked for us on several occasions and I was grateful.

Another question that may arise during an evaluation with a lactation specialist has to do with feeding schedules. After ten minutes of feeding, I told Pat that I was ready to put Tyler on the other breast. She asked me why. I told her that this is what I was told to do by the nurses at the hospital. They said to allow Tyler to feed the same amount of time on each breast for milk production reasons. I had no idea that this was misinformation. Most of the women I knew followed this same type of feeding schedule with only some variations in the amount of time spent on each breast.

Pat corrected this misinformation. She stated that if a breast is still full with milk, ideally, the mother should let the baby drink until the breast is fully drained. She explained that if the baby is still hungry after feeding on one breast, the mother should then transfer him to the other. If he is full and does not want to eat anymore, the mother can either pump the milk out of the full breast or wait until the next feeding and start him on that one.

The reason that this is preferable is because the baby will ultimately receive more nutritional value by draining one full breast instead of drinking only partially from both. There are two kinds of breast milk: foremilk and hindmilk. The foremilk is the milk that the baby first receives when latching onto the breast and feeding initially. It is not filled with the same level of fat or nutrients as hindmilk. It is even a different color, looking like watered-down cow's milk. In contrast, the hindmilk is high in fat and nutrients and is very important for a baby's health. It is thicker and has a more yellowish tone to it. It is this that allows the baby to feel full and content following a feeding.

The hindmilk can be obtained only after the foremilk is depleted. Therefore, if a mother changes breasts after only ten or fifteen minutes, the baby will probably not get any hindmilk and in turn could be much less satisfied after his feedings. In addition, if a baby falls asleep on the breast before getting to the hindmilk, he will probably not get what he needs in the way of calories and nutrition.

Pat instructed me to leave Tyler on the same breast until it felt like there was no more milk left inside of it. After another five minutes or so, I told her that I thought my breast was empty. She felt it and agreed that the milk was gone. She took Tyler from me and placed him back on the scale. I couldn't believe it. When Pat picked him up, he did not start crying. He was content in her arms and on the scale. This was a very new experience for me. I immediately noticed but didn't know what to say or do. In fact, there was nothing to do—for once!

I started Tyler on the other breast, but he did not feed much longer. He soon fell fast asleep. Since he consumed a lot of milk already, there was no reason to push him to stay awake. However, this circumstance provided us with the perfect opportunity to practice transferring him from the breast to a finger or a pacifier. I chose to go with my finger. Jason and I were pleasantly surprised that it worked so well. From that day forward, Tyler often sucked on one of our pinky fingers after feedings before drifting off to a deeper sleep. He sometimes enjoyed a pacifier, but this was not his preference. He definitely wanted to remain physically connected to us in some way. I often wondered if he too felt the same bonding moment that I did.

Allergies

One of the possible reasons that your baby simply won't stop crying is food allergies. Therefore, this is another important factor to consider when you are in the midst of assessment and diagnosis. I spoke with both my pediatrician and my lactation specialist about this possibility. Although food allergies are not totally uncommon in babies, they are not frequently seen among newborns either.

Parents with a colicky infant will usually not leave a single rock unturned when trying to find an answer to the perpetual crying in their home. Jason and I were no different. I investigated this possibility as I had all others. I did not want to take the chance of missing something that could be fixed so simply. Dealing with food allergies is in fact simple, however, it may not be easy.

There are two types of allergies to look for. The first is an allergy to the mother's breast milk. It is incredibly uncommon for babies to be allergic to their mother's breast milk. In contrast, it is much more common for babies to be allergic to a specific food ingredient such as dairy or wheat. This is the second type of allergy to investigate and should take precedence over the first unless your pediatrician advises you otherwise.

Interestingly, if you look at the statistics, it is not very common for babies to be allergic to specific food ingredients. Research shows that, in general, the prevalence of food allergies in children is 3 to 7 percent. More specifically, the prevalence of a dairy allergy is only 0.5 to 4 percent and a wheat allergy under 2 percent in infants. For both of these, the prevalence decreases with age. Babies who are suffering from a dairy or wheat allergy may voice their distress through crying.

Others may simply deal with it in silence. If a colicky baby has a food allergy, it is likely that his reaction will be the former of the two.

When exploring the possibility of food allergies, it is first important for breast-feeding mothers to be aware that whatever food they are consuming, their baby is consuming as well through their breast milk. In other words, if a breast-feeding mother is consuming foods that are high in protein, her baby is consuming foods that are high in protein; if a breast-feeding mother is consuming foods that are high in starch, her baby is consuming foods that are high in starch; and if a breast-feeding mother is consuming alcohol, her baby is consuming alcohol. This is important information because if your baby is intolerant to dairy or wheat and you are consuming those products, then your baby is consuming those products as well.

Babies can have all sorts of food intolerances. However, it is much more common for babies to be intolerant to dairy products than to wheat products. Therefore, if you are interested in investigating the possibility of food allergies, it is preferable to start with dairy and then move to wheat if no changes are found. In either case, there are only two options that you can pursue in order to fix this problem.

The first option entails an alteration in your diet. You will need to cut all dairy products out of your diet (and then wheat if necessary) including an ingredient found in many foods called *whey*. This means reading a lot of labels and making sure that nothing you consume includes these ingredients. You might be surprised at how many different foods actually include dairy products.

If you choose this option, it will mean making some potentially large changes in your eating habits. Therefore, you will need to prepare yourself and your family for this. That is not to say that if you cut out dairy products in your diet that everyone else will have to as well. However, it does mean a potential for more work placed on you with various new cooking demands. For example, you may end up cooking two meals for dinner rather than one meal for the whole family due to varying desires and requirements. I know the thought of placing more work on yourself when you are already overworked and overtired as a new parent sounds dreary. However, if your baby is intolerant to a certain food, it will be well worth the effort in the end.

You may already not be eating as well as you should be because of the lack of time you have to prepare nutritious meals with a colicky baby at home. For many parents with a colicky infant, nutritious food preparation is low on their priority list. Home-cooked meals are often replaced with take-out food. I know this was the case for Jason and me. We rarely ate take-out prior to Tyler's birth, but after he was born, it became common practice in our home. Therefore, I personally was not worried about an alteration in my diet. I figured it could not be worse than what I was already doing. However, other parents may be highly concerned. If you are one of these parents, consult with your doctor or with a nutritionist, especially if you have special dietary needs.

If you avoid dairy products and find that there is no change in your infant's crying pattern (i.e., a decrease in the amount or duration of crying around meals), then you can attempt to eliminate wheat products from your diet. I want to stress the importance again of eliminating dairy products first and wheat products second. It is highly important that you do not eliminate them both at the same time. If you do then you will never know to which one of them your baby is allergic. It is recommended to stick with this diet for one week. After that time, if there is no change it probably means that your baby is not dairy or wheat intolerant. Most women see a change within a twenty-four-hour period.

As I have discussed earlier, in order for you to find out what is affecting your infant so severely, you will have to try many different things. In essence, you will have to place yourselves in the role of detectives. Jason and I felt like we were playing detective ever since Tyler was born in order to find a cure to his colicky outbursts. In turn, altering my diet was not that different from the numerous strategies we had tried thus far. For me, although looking at labels and trying to plan meals would be a much more tedious process than before, it would be well worth it if food allergies were at the root of Tyler's problem.

Since Tyler did experience some digestive issues, Jason and I decided to go after the source instead of simply trying to remedy the problem. In other words, along with providing him with Mylicon drops and gripe water, I began a dairy-free diet, which lasted for over one week, and then began to cut wheat out of my diet as well. I was down to what I called "prison food." I basically ate rice and water three times per day. I found some decent breads and vegan muffins at an organic grocery store, which provided me with at least some diversity. I tried boiling chicken from time to time to get some better protein in my system, but without the ability to put any kind of sauce on it, the whole thing seemed pointless. Food was becoming less and less of a necessity.

I knew this could not be good for me nutritionally. I couldn't keep this diet up for long, but I was determined to see if it would provide Tyler with some relief. If you eliminate foods out of your diet in an attempt to find a solution, you should at minimum continue taking your prenatal vitamins.

Most individuals who are allergic to dairy or wheat products during infancy eventually outgrow their food intolerances; however, some do not. Unfortunately, there is no way of knowing for certain until the newborn is much older. One clue that may shed some light onto the probability of a food allergy is seeing if there is a family history of this problem. Find out if anyone in your family currently suffers or has suffered in the past—particularly during infancy—from a dairy or wheat allergy.

Research indicates that food allergies are often hereditary. I investigated this possibility in my own family during my search for answers. I learned that my paternal grandmother was not able to tolerate cow's milk when she was a baby. She could not hold it down. Her doctors were incredibly concerned about her severe weight loss during the first few weeks of her life due to this problem. Luckily, at the time her family owned a goat and her mother came up with the idea of giving her goat's milk instead. My grandmother is now ninety-one years old. During those times, they did not have the same options that we have today. Luckily, the idea to feed her goat's milk worked. It saved her life.

I also learned that my father was dairy intolerant. According to my grandmother, "He cried and cried after bottle-feedings." The cow's milk did not sit well with him either. Both my grandmother and my father are able to drink milk now and eventually outgrew this problem. However, my paternal aunt was not as lucky. She did not cry as an infant the way that my father did. However, she was recently diagnosed with lactose intolerance and never even knew she had this problem.

The second option that you have to fix the problem of a food allergy entails the cessation of breast-feeding, which means that you will need to begin bottle-feeding. There are two detriments to bottle-feeding. First, the infant will not receive the potential benefits of building his immune system if he is not breast-fed. Immunities from the mother are passed through her milk to her baby. Therefore, breast-fed babies tend to have a higher resistance to infection. This protection cannot be duplicated by formula. Second, the baby will not receive the same overall nutrition that is provided by the mother's milk. Breast milk is the ideal first food for you baby. However, most experts agree that the formulas made today are very different from the ones made in the past. They note that the similarity between formula and breast milk is almost identical now, and therefore, will not harm a baby due to lack of nutrition.

In addition, the cessation of breast-feeding eliminates the many benefits it provides to the mother. First, breast-feeding causes contractions to the uterus. After birth, the uterus contracts in order to shrink in size until it is the same as it was prepregnancy. This process takes approximately six weeks. Breast-feeding assists in this process after birth and helps avoid excessive bleeding. Second, breast-feeding burns calories. It is estimated that approximately 300 to 500 calories are burned each day by the breast-feeding mother. This can help the mother return more quickly to her prepregnancy weight. Third, it is economical. The added cost of formula can be burdensome for many families. Fourth, breast-feeding is more convenient. It is always ready on demand. There is nothing to prepare and it is always fresh and warm. Lastly, research indicates that breast-feeding may be helpful in lowering the risks of certain medical problems later in life, such as breast and uterine cancer.

If you choose to go the route of bottle-feeding, then selecting the best formula for your baby will be important. For example, if your baby is allergic to dairy products, then placing him on a formula that is free from dairy would solve the problem. Many parents try soy formulas first in an attempt to determine if their baby has a dairy intolerance. If there is no change in their baby's crying pattern, they then often try a formula called *Nutramigen* made by Enfamil. Nutramigen is easy to digest and specifically formulated to ease the discomfort of babies with gas and stomach upsets. It is marketed to help infants who have been diagnosed with colic.

There are some common problems associated with both formulas listed above. The most common problem with the soy formulas is that they often cause constipation in babies and can lead to great discomfort. The most common problem with Nutramigen is that it is highly expensive. Although this was good information to have when I was contemplating trying this option, I remember my largest concern was not with these common problems but rather with the potential downside of switching to formula at all. I spoke with both my lactation specialist and Tyler's pediatrician about my concerns in an attempt to decrease some of my fears.

Just as in the case of eliminating foods from your diet, switching from breast-feeding to bottle-feeding should yield results rather quickly. In fact, within a few days of this switch you should see a drastic change in your baby's distress level if he is indeed colicky from either a breast milk allergy or dairy intolerance. Most parents observe a difference right away (in the first twenty-four hours), however, to be certain you should try formula for at least one week.

As discussed previously, most parents try soy milk formula first. This formula tastes very different than breast milk, so be prepared for your baby to initially reject it. He will have to adjust to the taste difference. This adjustment takes different amounts of time according to the varying needs of the infant. Some babies may take to the new formula right away and others may reject it several times before accepting it as their only source of food.

If your baby rejects formula, one helpful tip is to initially mix your breast milk and formula together. This will create a smoother transition to formula feedings for your infant. Start out with a bottle filled predominantly with breast milk and only some formula. At each successive feeding, you should slowly increase the amount of formula in the bottle as you slowly decrease the amount of breast milk. If you utilize this process, it will take longer to see if your baby is dairy intolerant, but it may ease the shock of the transition and provide him with less confusion and distress.

Tyler was accustomed to breast milk and was somewhat resistant to the change. We tried the soy milk formula first. Luckily, he eventually gave in and drank it. Unfortunately, within forty-eight hours, we had to discontinue its use. It caused horrible constipation for him, which caused him further distress. He did not poop once while consuming this product. We then switched to the Nutramigen formula for colicky infants. We knew this formula was extremely expensive but that many parents found it to be useful because it was so easy for infants to digest. Although the expense was a concern, we were willing to find a way as long as it worked.

Jason and I joked with each other that we would pay a thousand dollars a day for a formula that worked. Does it sound like we were desperate? Well, we were. Putting all joking aside however, the reality for many parents is that they cannot afford an expensive formula for their infants. If you are one of these parents, do not disregard this alternative solely due to the cost. There are creative ways to obtain this formula affordably if indeed this is what your baby needs.

First, call your pediatrician to inform him that you are going to try Nutramigen in an attempt to solve colic and ask him for some free samples. This is a good idea for anyone who would like to attempt its use so that you won't have to incur the costs of the formula if it does not work. This formula is approximately two and a half times the cost of others. Our pediatrician's exact words were: "You could pay for your child's college tuition with the money you will spend on this formula in a year." Second, try contacting the manufacturer, Enfamil, and ask if they would be willing to donate some cans to you. I know one woman who had twins. Both of her babies were colicky and the only formula that worked for them was Nutramigen. Their mother talked with the manufacturer and received several free cases of formula from the company. It saved a large amount of money.

When Jason and I switched Tyler to Nutramigen, he once again had to adjust to a new taste. He was resistant at first, but eventually drank it. The Nutramigen did not cause constipation. In contrast, it was easy for him to digest and his excretion pattern was back on track. Almost everyone I spoke with and almost everything I read about Nutramigen indicated that if a baby is allergic to his mother's breast milk or allergic to some specific food allergy, once placed on this formula, the change will be almost instantaneous. Several women who I talked to online noted that they saw changes within a twenty-four hour period. Unfortunately, I was not one of them.

Another week went by and still nothing changed. At the end of this week, Tyler turned two and a half months old. After seven days of being solely bottle-fed with the Nutramigen, Jason and I came to the conclusion that this was not going to relieve Tyler's discomfort. Like everything else so far, it helped, but did not provide us with a cure. Still we did not get frustrated. I was convinced that there was something out there that would relieve my son's distress and was motivated to find it.

If you decide to try formula feedings in attempt to give your baby some relief, you will need to prepare for the possibility that it may not work. One important preparation is to utilize a breast pump in the absence of breast-feeding. Unless you are planning to give up breast-feeding all together during this experimental stage, it is wise to pump your breast milk during formula feedings. This is important so that your body continues to produce the same amount of milk necessary to meet your baby's needs. Remember, breast milk is produced in the body under the supply-and-demand theory. Therefore, the cessation of breast-feedings with no pumping will eventually result in a depleted milk supply. Most women choose to keep their milk supply up in case they decide to go back to breast-feeding if this option fails. This is exactly what I chose to do, and I was glad because it did indeed fail.

I was very lucky that Tyler allowed me to go back to breast-feeding. After two weeks of only bottle-feedings, he could have easily rejected the breast. However, he did not. He took to the breast as if he had never left it. Other parents may not be so lucky. If your infant rejects the breast after he has been bottle-fed for a designated period of time, you ultimately have only two choices. You can either stick with bottle-feedings or persevere in your attempts to get him back onto the breast. If you choose the latter and are struggling with this attempt, contact a lactation specialist for guidance, advice, and support.

I was glad to have the breast-feeding bonding time with my son again. I did not realize how much I missed it when I was bottle-feeding him until I resumed the breast-feeding process. Although he was content with the bottle, there was no physical joining between the two of us when he was bottle-fed. I missed that connection. After all, it was one of the only connections I had during his stormy days of colic.

Some parents choose not to switch back to breast-feeding completely. Instead, they continue to bottle-feed their baby from time to time for a variety of reason. First, it can provide other family members, particularly the other parent, with some baby bonding time as well. Second, it can give the mother a break in the middle of the night. Nighttime feedings can be exhausting when only one parent is in charge of them. This is especially true if a baby requires more frequent feedings. Third, many mothers plan to go back to work and want their baby to stay familiar with the bottle so that he will not have to make this difficult transition later. Experts recommend introducing the bottle early on (often in the first few months of life) to get the baby accustomed to bottle-feedings. They note that the longer you wait, the harder the adjustment will be for the baby.

Whatever option or options you choose to help your baby relieve his distress, you will inevitably be met with challenges along the way. Let's face it, if the choice was simple, there would be no options and there would be no need to choose. The reason that the choice is not simple is because your baby is unique. Therefore, be prepared to try all options before deciding what works best for him.

I will reiterate the point that during this process, you really will feel like you are doing investigative work. Most parents try out all of the tips and suggestions they gain from experts who know something about colic. If the suggested strategies that you receive do not work, you will need to move onto the next ones. The reality is that some will work for you and some will not. Unfortunately, there is no science that tells us what will work for one baby and not for another. As a parent of a colicky infant, you become the scientist for your baby and your attempts become the science.

Lastly, I would like to note that during my family's search to find answers, Jason and I often joked with one another that it was almost as if the pediatricians and lactation specialists conspired together to keep parents of colicky infants hopeful. I think most parents with a colicky infant would agree that they thankfully provide suggestions and offer action plans to overwhelmed parents who are looking to find some relief. In my experience, many parents have also agreed that these suggestions and action plans often last just long enough until the colic runs its course and cures itself. Maybe this is in hope that parents will find a cure. Sometimes this occurs. However, as time went on, Jason and I became more and more convinced that it was for the main purpose of keeping parents sane. Nothing is worse than feeling hopeless. (See Chapter 6, "Living with a Nightmare," for information on how to cope with the distress of colic.)

CHAPTER REVIEW

Pediatrician

Tips

* Make an in-office appointment so that your pediatrician can directly observe the problem of colic.
* Schedule the appointment during the time that your infant will most likely be colicky.

Initial Strategies

* Vibration.
* White noise.
* Water therapy.
* Infant massage.

Infant GERD or Gassiness

* In order for these to be properly diagnosed, your pediatrician will need information about your baby's crying patterns.
* Be prepared to give him a detailed description of when your baby cries and for how long.
* If an individual suffers from GERD then it means that acid and other stomach contents repeatedly flow back up into the esophagus.
* The most common symptoms of infant GERD are: (1) frequent or recurrent vomiting, (2) frequent or persistent cough, and (3) heartburn, gas, or abdominal pain.
* Under certain circumstances your pediatrician may request additional tests to ascertain the problem.

* Infant GERD is not difficult to diagnose but is often left undiagnosed due to a variety of reasons.
* There are specific treatment interventions for infant GERD that have been proven successful, such as alteration in feeding and sleeping position, medication, and in more severe cases, surgery.

Lactation Specialist

Reason for Consultation
* To assess for proper latch onto the breast.
* To assess the mother's milk supply.
* To obtain accurate information about breast-feeding.

What to Expect
* Most consultation sessions will involve an evaluation of the mother breast-feeding her baby through behavioral observation.
* Before the evaluation begins, the lactation specialist will weigh the baby. This is done to establish a baseline weight, which will be compared to the baby's weight following the feeding session.
* A lactation specialist may request a physical evaluation of your breast in an assessment to see if it is full of milk before you begin the feeding and empty once the feeding is complete.
* During the evaluation, your lactation specialist will most likely engage you in conversation and ask direct questions about breast-feeding positions, technique, and schedules.

What You'll Learn
* How to assure proper latch onto the breast and reduce sore nipples.

* How to keep the baby awake while breast-feeding.
* How to transition the baby from the breast to the bed without waking him.
* The importance of hindmilk versus foremilk.

Food Allergies

* A food allergy may be one of the possible reasons that your baby simply won't stop crying.
* There are two types of allergies to look for: an allergy to the mother's breast milk or an allergy to a specific food ingredient, such as dairy or wheat.
* Food allergies are uncommon among infants and they usually outgrow them with time.
* For breast-feeding mothers, treatment options include an alteration in diet or the cessation of breast-feeding.
* Bottle-feeding suggestions and how to choose the right formula for your baby.
* How to prepare for the fact that bottle-feedings may not cure the colic symptoms.
* Prepare yourself that with whatever option or options you choose to help your baby relieve his distress, you will inevitably be met with challenges along the way.

Chapter 5

Finally an Answer

If you are one of the many people who are struggling currently with a colicky infant, my guess is that you skipped directly to this chapter to find a quick solution. Good for you! Getting some relief is the key to survival when faced with colic. I've listed specific strategies that, through time and with better understanding, helped my family and thousands of others survive the many months of colic.

Background

When Tyler was three and a half months old, his colic was not yet gone. I have to admit I was frustrated, even though I was beginning to see a change in his behavior for the better. Things were not nearly as bad as they were in the first three months. However, Tyler was still in distress a lot of the time. Furthermore, his crying, although not nearly as frequent and severe, was still present throughout much of the day. I began to doubt the colic would ever stop.

As mentioned in previous chapters, contrary to what many people had told us, Tyler did not experience an abrupt cessation of his colic symptoms at one hundred days. Remember, this is the date that an infant's digestive system is fully developed and therefore, struggles with "tummy troubles" are supposed to magically disappear. I have actually heard women tell me that when their colicky infant turned one hundred days old, "The difference was like night and day." This was not true in our case and unfortunately, it is not true for many.

For us, the symptoms gradually decreased with time. Tyler's colic was more severe than most from the beginning, and he was not going to be one of the easier cases in the end. Perhaps this is what drove my obsession to search for answers and find a cure. Finding answers was very difficult. One of my biggest frustrations was that what worked for many infants did not work for Tyler. Every infant is different. Thus the key is to find out what is driving the colic and then to figure out the best strategy to soothe the baby.

As discussed in Chapter 1, "Theories of Colic," in order to treat a problem effectively, you must first identify the cause of the problem. I believe this is what makes colic so hard to treat. One only sees a drastic "night and day" change when a specific medical cause can be associated with the colic—for instance "big tummy troubles" such as acid reflux, which can be treated with medication, or "little tummy troubles" such as gas or constipation, which can be treated with over-the-counter medications or home remedies. (See Chapter 4, "Treatment Approaches for Specific Causes".)

Most cases of colic have no discernable medical cause that can be directly linked to the onset and continuance of this problem. Therefore, it is imperative to find answers in the realm of psychology. Learning how to calm the infant who is unable to self-soothe, and finding ways to teach him these self-soothing techniques, is imperative in finding some relief. Taking care of yourself in the process is paramount, but not a priority for most. We are about to change that. Chapter 7 focuses on how to take care of the caregiver.

Resources

There are very few resources for the caregiver of the colicky infant. Since I went through emotional and physical struggles myself, I was aware that even if there were an abundance of resources to help, there would be very little time to utilize them. Every day that my son screamed relentlessly, I fantasized about gaining the knowledge and skill to soothe him. Having an easy, concrete, and understandable guide describing interventions that I could try to calm my child would have been a godsend. This is why I am including it in this book for the countless parents who are currently standing in my shoes.

There are very few books on the market that prescribe how to treat colic. When searching for "colic" in a literature review, almost all of the books that are listed are either out of print or focus on equine colic. It seems absurd that there are more books on horse colic than human colic; nonetheless, this is the case. In my own search for answers, I expanded my search to the more general topic of "crying babies." Not surprisingly, hundreds of books came up in this baby category. Some of these books offered a small subsection on colic; however, most did not touch upon the subject at all. Furthermore, there was not a single book that focused on the complete package of colic assessment, diagnosis, and intervention, coupled with the emotions that individuals face when struggling with this problem.

If you have a colicky infant, you have probably heard many times by now, "There is no cure for colic" and "You will simply have to wait it out." I cannot count the amount of times that Jason and I heard these words while we were searching for answers. Luckily, neither one of us was willing to believe that *nothing* could be done to help our situation. Each time I heard these words, I wondered how parents manage to wait three months for crying to stop on its own without being able to console their baby and keep from going completely insane. After all, we live in a world of technology and scientific research far beyond what individuals who lived before us could have ever imagined. It seemed almost impossible not to have a cure for something as basic as a child's relentless screaming.

A Theory on Colic That Makes Sense

Many pediatric experts report that when a baby enters the world, he or she is confronted with stimulation that can be incredibly overwhelming and often distressing. After all, the newborn has lived in protected comfort for over nine months in utero. The newborn is not familiar with the sights, sounds, tastes, smells, and touch that envelop him the moment that he is born. Imagine how the newborn must feel when he first enters the world faced with so many changes.

Instinctively, many of these newborns find ways to shut out the rest of the world and the overstimulation that they are ultimately forced to experience. For example, most babies when overstimulated will sleep. This is their coping mechanism. It is one of the few things that they have control over at such a young age. These infants have found a way to calm themselves and to self-soothe.

Unfortunately, some babies are not able to self-soothe as easily. They cannot shut out the world and need some help to do so. These babies communicate their distress in the only way that they know how: through crying. Unfortunately, hearing their own cries is distressing and overstimulating in itself. This becomes a self-perpetuating cycle of uncontrollable and relentless crying. As mentioned earlier, it is important to remember that crying is the infant's form of self-expression.

The newborn is basically saying that he is feeling overwhelmed or overstimulated and does not know how to fix it.

Colicky infants may notice everything around them. Tyler was this way. He paid attention to every detail, which in turn led to his over-stimulation. I remember when Tyler was under one month old; he effortlessly tracked objects that were within view. People around Tyler would comment, "He is so alert at such a young age!" This advanced developmental milestone is precisely what leads to the infant becoming overwhelmed. Being jolted with stimuli coupled with an inability to self-soothe is exactly what leads to colic. In other words, for an infant to suffer from colic that is not caused by medical problems, he must be highly reactive to stimuli and have an inability to calm or self-soothe.

My son fit both of these criteria. In addition to being highly responsive to stimuli, Tyler has never been able to self-soothe. I remember thinking about his struggles in the context of other babies that I have observed through the years. I thought about the numerous times that I have been to social gatherings and have seen babies sleeping amongst tremendous amounts of noise. I always wondered how they could do that. Tyler never could. Tyler would be awake and screaming under those circumstances every single time. Babies who sleep through these situations are shutting out the stimulation around them so that they will not feel overwhelmed.

Being highly sensitive to stimuli and not being able to self-soothe becomes viewed as part, if not all, of a baby's temperament. In my literature review, I read that colicky infants are often very smart. Perhaps it is because they are inquisitive and pay attention to detail. This attention to stimulation was the one cause of colic that seemed to really fit for Tyler. It may also be the one that fits for your baby, especially if he is not crying due to gastrointestinal problems.

If this cause does seem to fit your infant, then it means your baby's temperament plays a large role in determining his colic. It is common for a baby to inherit the trait of temperament from one or both of his parents. I knew that my temperament was very different from Tyler's; however, I saw resemblances in temperament between Tyler and Jason. For example, Tyler is a hard-to-soothe baby who notices every change in his environment. He is incredibly sensitive to the stimuli around him, which is why when there is a change in his environment he notices immediately. He reacts to sound, sight, smell, taste, and touch. Jason is the same way. Jason has never been a good sleeper or a good self-soother. Jason also notices everything that goes on around him and reacts to it. Nothing gets past either one of them.

I remember contacting Jason's family to inquire about his family history. Jason was also a colicky infant. His parents noted that he was never as bad off as Tyler was, but he was often crying as an infant and was very difficult to soothe. They noted that the hardest part for them was that Jason was not a good sleeper. According to Jason's father, "He wore us down." He would often be up until 11:00 p.m. at night (way past their bedtime) and then be up at 5:00 a.m. the next morning. Jason's father recalled that on certain nights they would pad all the walls in Jason's room with pillows to make it baby safe and leave him in there to play until he finally fell asleep. At midnight they would find him asleep on the floor and put him in his crib. Upon hearing this, I wondered if this is what we had in store for us in the future with Tyler. After all, sleep patterns can be genetic as well.

The Answer

Through time and reading I learned that the best way to calm your colicky infant is what most caregivers do intuitively without even realizing it. The feelings of hopelessness and helplessness that result from constant inconsolable infant crying often prevent caregivers from recognizing that their interventions and efforts *do indeed work*. Instead, the caregiver *gives up too quickly* before gaining at least some success in calming their infant.

For example, when a baby cries most parents instinctively pick the baby up, draw him close to their body, and say "shhhhhh." They then begin to sing or talk to him softly as they glide around the room in a swaying motion. If these strategies do not work, most parents become creative and invent their own techniques that may calm their child. One of my close friends did "a rain dance" every time his daughter became fussy at night. Another one of my friends swaddled her baby tight, turned on music and held her close to her body as she practiced her marching band routine in the living room; it worked every time.

Below is a list of some of the most common published ways to soothe a colicky infant. Interestingly, when speaking with caregivers who have struggled with colic, almost all of them state that the strategies listed below are ones that they have at one time or another tried. Some attempts were successful and some were not. The ones that were not were often never tried again. It is important to recognize that your attempt to calm your infant may not have been successful simply because it was given up too soon.

Five Specific Methods

Several experts in the field who have published bestselling books (i.e., Dr. Harvey Karp, *The Happiest Baby on the Block* and Tracy Hogg with Melinda Blau, *Secrets of the Baby Whisperer*) have cited specific methods to accomplish the task of soothing a newborn. These methods can be applied to difficult babies as well as colicky infants.

Method 1: The Baby Swaddle

In utero babies are held in a small space without the ability to flail their arms and legs around the way they can once they are born. This tight, secure hold is comfortable and safe for them. If a baby is swaddled correctly (with an inability to break out of the hold), then he will once again feel comfort, safety, and security, which is exactly what he became accustomed to in his first nine months. This method has been around for centuries.

In the past, before women went to hospitals to deliver their babies, midwives came into their home to assist with labor and delivery. During these times, after the birth, the midwife swooped the baby away to be swaddled in a blanket before presenting him to his mother. Today, most mothers have the opportunity to meet their newborn first before they are whisked off by nurses who clean and wrap the baby in the comfort of their first baby blanket. Jason and I learned how to swaddle Tyler in the hospital. It was the very first strategy that we attempted intuitively when Tyler began to cry.

I believe that caregivers instinctively wrap their babies as a way to protect them from an array of environmental forces. For example, it is not uncommon for parents to wrap their infant in a blanket as a way to keep him snug and warm. Also, by wrapping an infant in a blanket, you are indirectly keeping him protected from others. The baby is less vulnerable with this shield wrapped around. How many parents do you know—and maybe you are one of them—who do not like it when others try to touch their newborns? Perhaps this is for good reason (e.g., worry about catching germs, discomfort with strangers who attempt to invade personal space, etc.). Regardless of the reasons, it is human nature to protect your young. The swaddle is the first thing taught to provide this protection and is available from the beginning.

Method 2: Placing the Baby on His Stomach or on His Side

Babies are not used to being placed on their backs. In fact, when they are held in this position, they experience the Moro reflex. The Moro reflex is when the infant feels as if he is falling. This experience can be extremely distressful for a baby. The baby will flail his arms about as if trying to catch himself from a fall when this occurs.

Adults experience the Moro reflex as well, often as they are drifting off to sleep. Their bodies twitch so severely that the twitching wakes the individual up. Feeling as if you are falling backwards can be very unsettling for adults. Imagine how much more unsettling this might be for an infant who is new to the world.

Placing an infant on his stomach or on his side will prevent him from experiencing the Moro reflex (by the way, the same is true for adults). This strategy is utilized by many caregivers. Perhaps this is because many caregivers were raised by parents who provided this sleeping and playing position for them. I know lying on my stomach was my primary sleep position for the majority of my infancy and childhood.

As I am sure most of you are very aware, the reason for the shift in sleep position from stomach to back stems from occurrences of SIDS (sudden infant death syndrome). Due to the reality of SIDS, I feel compelled to note that parents will need to be watchful and attentive to their child if they choose to utilize this technique. Doctors highly recommend that babies sleep on their back and not on their stomach. The side position seems to be becoming more popular as a compromise; especially with the many safety devices now being sold in baby stores, which promise to hold the infant in place so that there is little risk of him rolling over onto his stomach.

Method 3: White Noise

This sound mimics the sound of the blood flow in utero. White noise can be created for the newborn in many different ways. In its most basic or simplistic form, it is the shushing sound often made by a caregiver when an infant is crying. Many individuals have created white noise by turning their radio or TV on to a station that only has static. White noise has become such a popular calming strategy that once again the baby market is filled with devices that create this noise. For example, as mentioned in an earlier chapter, Jason and I bought a baby sound machine that provided white noise. This machine had volume control and a timer attached which allowed the white noise to turn off at a fifteen-, thirty-, or sixty-minute intervals. Jason and I were familiar with the white noise intervention in dealing with Tyler. We placed the white noise machine in Tyler's room at night. This helped somewhat, but was not a miracle cure.

Jason and I tried shushing in Tyler's ear every time he became fussy. It seemed the natural thing to do. Perhaps this technique is learned from others. I know that most parents do this when their baby cries. However, I believe that it is pure instinct for a mother to want to calm her child and the "shhhhhh" sound is what has been used for centuries. Even though the shushing alone did not often work for Tyler, it was a strategy I used throughout his colicky months.

I have to admit, I was excited the day that, by accident, I stumbled onto a way to utilize this strategy more successfully. In the midst of utter frustration after a long sleepless night with Tyler screaming relentlessly, I could not take his crying anymore. I felt like I was losing my mind. I wanted to scream out loud and at him. It took every ounce of effort not to. Instead, I began shushing in his ear, but this did not work. On this occasion, instead of giving up like I usually did, I shushed louder. Tyler was screaming so loud, I could not even hear my own shushing, so I naturally did what any sleep-deprived, frustrated parent would do—I shushed louder. It became a battle of who could scream the loudest and my shushing was my scream. Interestingly, and almost unbelievably, this seemed to calm Tyler down. It occurred to me that maybe he could not hear my shushing over his loud cries.

This is a wonderful example of how parents often give up too easily with the strategies that they intuitively attempt with their infants. If I had not persisted, I would not have found something that helped to calm my child. Caregivers need to shush loud enough and long enough to calm their crying infant. If you think about this it makes sense. If a colicky infant is in the midst of a relentless screaming session he is not going to hear the soft shushing noise provided by his parent.

The thought of this made me laugh. It was not easy to shush louder than Tyler's blood-curdling screams. I was worried that if I continued to utilize this strategy I would end up hyperventilating and passing out. But what other choice did I have? How in the world could Tyler hear me if I was gently shushing in his ear? I could barely hear myself over his loud cries.

Many experts note that most parents wrongly assume that their newborns prefer soft, gentle sounds. It seems counterintuitive that they would prefer the opposite. However, we have to remember that this is what babies are used to. For nine months they heard the loud sound of blood flowing through their mother's body. This noise was constant and continual and also extremely soothing.

Method 4: Movement

Movement is a highly marketed intervention to soothe a fussy infant. When you walk into a baby store, there are aisles full of baby devices that provide the baby with some form of motion. Vibrating chairs, baby swings, jumpers, and rockers, are all advertised to calm the fussy infant. Although the baby industry has capitalized on this idea, intuitively caregivers have provided their infants with movement for centuries: walking, bouncing, or swaying.

Infants are used to movement in utero. Whenever the mother moved, the baby could feel it. Therefore, swinging infants back and forth recreates what they were used to for nine months. This movement is very soothing for them. Before we understood the true reasoning behind this, Jason and I had a standing joke about its usefulness. Tyler was conceived when we were on a vacation where I spent hours daily on a flying trapeze. We joked that he became used to the swinging motion before I even knew I was pregnant.

Swinging Tyler was one thing that helped us with him tremendously. The swinging method we employed was our saving grace. It allowed us to build the confidence to go places, see people, and return some normalcy to our lives. We simply reminded each other that if we ran into a problem, we could always swing Tyler to calm and soothe him and things would be okay.

We started going to Jason's softball games, over to friends' houses, the mall, the supermarket, etc. I am sure that some people must have thought we were crazy for swinging Tyler in his car seat for extended periods of time, but we did what worked. Many of our friends asked if they could help and it felt good to let them take a turn. However, I have to admit that it felt even better when they would stop swinging him to take a rest and he would start wailing again. They would ask, "How do you do it? I am exhausted after five minutes." We would reply, "Welcome to our world."

That is exactly what it had become. Our own little world of managing a colicky infant—and we were getting good at it. However, we still had our struggles. There were times when Jason and I were so exhausted that we couldn't see straight. Sometimes the swinging alone didn't work and we had no other alternatives. Furthermore, the swinging was starting to take a toll on our bodies. The muscles in our shoulders and back were sore and inflamed. We kept reminding ourselves to take turns so neither one of us would pull something. If that happened, then we would really be in trouble.

Method 5: Sucking

Sucking is probably the most natural soothing technique for an infant and the one that the infant does himself instinctively. This self-soothing technique begins in utero for the baby when he learns how to suck his thumb. Interestingly, not only does the infant suck to nourish himself, but he sucks to learn about his world. An infant puts things in his mouth at a specific developmental stage to make sense of the objects around him. He learns about different shapes, sizes, textures, and tastes when sucking on a variety of objects.

Furthermore, sucking provides the infant and caregiver with an opportunity to bond. Whether the baby is breast or bottle-fed, a connection between caregiver and baby is formed. I believe that this is why several fathers comment on their enjoyment of bottle-feeding their newborn. It gives them a way to bond and connect with their baby that is similar to the mother's way. A father told me, "Our baby cried so much, the only time he was calm was when my wife fed him. I felt like I was missing out on a special time with my daughter. It was not until I started bottle-feeding her that I understood how important those moments were for them. I enjoyed sharing peaceful times with her too."

Sucking can take many forms. Newborns may suck while they are breast-feeding, bottle-feeding, or using a pacifier. They may also adopt the strategy of sucking on their thumb or hand. In any case, the sucking calms the newborn. Not only does it remind the infant of being in the womb, but it releases natural chemicals in the brain, which leads to deep relaxation. In addition, it is very hard for an infant to scream if he has something in his mouth. Therefore, sucking can provide numerous solutions to the relentless crying of the colicky infant.

As I have indicated before, one of the only times Tyler was content was while he was breast-feeding. Many babies like pacifiers. Tyler rarely did, but he did like sucking on my pinky finger. Later, a bottle was used to help soothe him. In fact, in Tyler's case, it was difficult to wean him from the bottle because it was one of the only things that he could engage in to soothe himself.

Best Chances for Success

I have already mentioned that what works to help soothe a colicky infant is what most caregivers do intuitively without even realizing it. However, the feelings of hopelessness and helplessness that result from constant, inconsolable infant crying often prevent caregivers from recognizing that their interventions and efforts do indeed work. Instead, the caregiver gives up too quickly before gaining at least some success in calming the infant. The biggest encouragement I can give to parents who are currently struggling with a colicky infant is not to give up too quickly. Prolonged exposure to self-soothing techniques often provides the infant with the learning experience he or she needs in order to utilize the technique offered.

Think about a time when you recently had to learn a new task. If someone was teaching you this new task and after only a few minutes gave up trying because clearly you had difficulty understanding what to do, how would you respond? If your answer is with frustration, anger, or helplessness, you would not be alone. Now imagine your infant, who is faced with this same struggle. Remember colicky infants are not able to self-soothe. Unlike other infants, they need to be taught how to calm themselves and it is the caregiver's job to teach them. If the caregiver gives up too quickly, then the baby will not learn and will be faced with the same feelings noted above which will inevitably lead to more crying.

Research indicates that in order to achieve success in calming the infant, a combination of methods may need to be employed at the same time. I believe that most caregivers intuitively attempt the various methods listed above, however, I do not believe that they intuitively attempt to combine the methods. Utilizing methods together may bring greater success. This makes sense if you think about it. Try applying this idea to yourself for example. Think about what soothes you as an adult.

I know that many individuals take hot baths to soothe themselves. Taking a hot bath might provide peace for that individual. However, adding some scented bubble bath to the water (aromatherapy), turning on some relaxing music, and lighting some candles may lead to even greater peace and serenity. In other words, one strategy for relaxation may result in relaxation, but several strategies used in combination could result in a much deeper relaxed state.

Jason and I learned that combining strategies was more helpful than utilizing one at a time. Swinging Tyler, breast-feeding him, white noise, swaddling him, and putting him on his side were all things that we tried at one time or another and found to helpful to varying degrees. However, we never tried them all together. It never occurred to us that doing them at the same time might be more effective. Finally, we began to combine the strategies we intuitively had been trying for months.

One day when Tyler was in the midst of one of his severe colicky episodes, I swaddled him in a blanket and began loudly shushing in his ear. As I was doing this, I turned him on his side and held him in my arms while I rocked him forward and backwards (not side to side because remember this movement is not what the infant is used to). At first Tyler was angry at being confined and screamed louder than he did before, but I did not give up. Tyler began to calm down. I couldn't believe it. I was so excited that I even tried to give him a pacifier to include the sucking technique, but Tyler wouldn't take it. However, it didn't matter. Tyler was much more content than he was before. In fact, after approximately ten minutes, he drifted off to sleep.

I wish I could say that this technique always worked. Unfortunately, it did not. But it did help. Perhaps more important, it gave me some hope that I would be able to help my son when in distress. In addition, I knew I was beginning to teach my son how to self-soothe. My actions replaced my words as I attempted to soothe him.

If we as caregivers could verbally communicate with the colicky baby about how to self-soothe, then life would undoubtedly be easier on everyone who is involved. Unfortunately, we cannot teach the colicky infant how to self-soothe with words, but we can nonverbally teach them through our actions. We can show them what needs to occur in order for them to calm themselves.

In reality, there is probably no single cause of colic, but rather a combination of factors that lead to this problem. When a baby enters the world, he is confronted with stimulation that can be incredibly overwhelming and often distressing to him. Instinctively, many of these newborns find ways to shut out the overstimulation they are experiencing. Unfortunately, colicky babies cannot and need help in learning to do so.

Learning how to calm the infant who is unable to self-soothe and finding ways to teach him these self-soothing techniques is imperative to finding some relief. Most caregivers intuitively utilize the published strategies to soothe a fussy infant without even realizing it. However, the feelings of hopelessness and helplessness that result from caring for a colicky infant often prevent caregivers from recognizing that prolonging and combining their interventions and efforts can work. The two biggest mistakes that caregivers make in their attempts to calm their colicky infant are: (1) giving up too quickly, and (2) only utilizing one method at a time. A combination of methods has been proven to be much more successful.

I have spent a lot of time discussing the emotional repercussions faced by individuals who are caring for a colicky infant. It is vitally important for the caregiver to care for himself or herself. This is true for any individual who is caring for a child. It is even more true for the parents of extremely colicky babies who are filled with emotions that leave them frustrated, angry, and doubting themselves as parents. Remember there is hope, and you and your baby will survive!

CHAPTER REVIEW

A Theory on Colic That Makes Sense
* Newborns are confronted with stimulation that can be incredibly overwhelming and often distressing.
* Instinctively, many of these newborns find ways to cope with this overstimulation by finding ways to self-soothe.
* Unfortunately, colicky babies are unable to self-soothe.
* Colicky infants notice everything around them.
* Being highly responsive to stimuli and being unable to self-soothe can together lead to colic.

The Answer
* The best way to calm your colicky infant is what most caregivers do intuitively without even realizing it.
* The biggest reason soothing techniques fail is because the parent gives up on his or her attempt too quickly.

Five Specific Methods
* The baby swaddle.
* Placing the baby on his stomach or on his side.
* White noise.
* Movement.
* Sucking.

Best Chances for Success
* Don't give up too easily or quickly with any given strategy.
* A combination of methods may need to be employed at the same time.

* Remind yourself that your baby is crying as a way to communicate with you.

Chapter 6

Living with a Nightmare

One of the most difficult things to do when someone is suffering from a chronic problem is to learn how to live with it. If you know anyone that suffers from a chronic illness, you know how devastating this can be for him and for those who care about him. Even though learning how to cope with a chronic problem will never lead to a cure, it can at least provide the individual and his loved ones with some relief.

Colic is a chronic problem. It may not be as long-lived as other chronic problems, but nonetheless the relentless, inconsolable cries of a newborn day after day, month after month, can be devastating to all those involved.

Preparation

One way to cope with a chronic problem is to know what to expect. This is often difficult to master when you have a colicky infant, due to his unpredictability. However, even if he is unpredictable, you do not have to be. Setting up some sort of schedule or daily routine can be extremely helpful when dealing with the inconsistent world of colic.

Several seasoned parents talk about making the transition to parenthood and how once a schedule and routine is in place things get easier. Many people do well with structure. Perhaps you are one of them. The question is: How do you get your baby on a schedule and set up a daily routine in your household? Many first-time parents don't even know what a baby's schedule is supposed to look like. In addition, they have been told that a baby usually makes his own schedule at a very young age. Although this may be true, many experts believe that you can set your baby's schedule and create a pattern that works for you.

Tyler had no pattern whatsoever. He slept when he slept, ate when he ate, and cried when he cried with changes all the time. It was next to impossible to set up a schedule for him. Although I attempted to do so and followed several experts' advice, most of my attempts were futile. I learned through my struggles that when you have a severely colicky infant, you cannot follow the ordinary rules of logic or advice. For example, I remember one expert recommending that you wake your infant at the same time each day to feed and play with him. Since Tyler did not nap at the same time each day (even with my attempts to let him "cry it out" in his crib), waking him up at the same time each day or after a specified amount of time would result in lack of sleep at best (sometimes he was playing catch up from the night before when he screamed for ten consecutive hours), and the initiation of another long colicky outburst at worst.

I spent a lot of time searching for answers on how to successfully create a schedule for my colicky infant. Unfortunately, I never found guidelines that worked. My conclusion was to do the best I could with what I had and what I knew about my son. He did not follow a given schedule until he was much older and I found validation from others who walked in my shoes with their own colicky infants and attested to the same struggles.

One way that I learned to cope with the chronic problem of colic was to take nothing for granted. I reveled in the joys of parenthood when I had them. As difficult as it was to have a colicky infant who cried sixteen hours a day, almost every day for six months, I did have some precious moments with my son. For example, I felt pure and utter joy with Tyler while breast-feeding.

Tyler was always content on the breast. This is one of the reasons I knew he did not suffer from infant GERD. I was happier and more content during this time as well. I would like to say that this solely occurred because my son was at peace with himself and that it was our best bonding time together, and although these two points are true, there is a physiological reason as well. Breast-feeding triggers the release of a hormone called prolactin. This hormone is often referred to as the "mothering hormone." This hormone is known to promote a feeling of calm relaxation, peacefulness, and overall well-being.

Psychological Ramifications to the Parent

When faced with unexpected challenges and forced to deal with a situation that is less than ideal, a person often feels anxious, confused, overwhelmed, and stressed. Many parents who have a colicky infant wonder why they have been chosen to confront the issue of colic. Unfortunately, there is no definitive answer. Parents will respond in varying ways to the difficulties set forth in caring for and raising a colicky infant. With this situation comes some psychological ramifications to the parent that I will discuss.

I have treated many patients on matters both realized and imagined. I am never surprised that people are confronted by intense emotional challenges. More important, I am heartened that they seek tools to combat them. One universal common denominator is the basic concept of struggling. This is indeed one of the most human elements that knows no bias. Parents who have a colicky infant often experience an array of emotions. Some are easier to admit and verbalize and some less so. It is the emotions that are seen as negative and difficult to express that concern me the most in my profession. I know how important it is to talk about difficult and sometimes devastating emotions. Without this discussion and exploration, these emotions can cause the greatest psychological ramifications and detriment.

My family's experience with colic was different than what we were told by various medical professionals and what we had read about in books. Every time Tyler was awake, he was crying relentlessly in full force. He stopped crying only to eat and sleep and sometimes for brief moments when he could be distracted by someone or something. As we experienced it, it was not an evening affair, but an all-day affair. The constant cries were not only unpleasant, they were traumatic. Like any other trauma, we experienced a form of post-traumatic stress due to the cries.

If parents of a colicky infant described their reaction to their infant's distress as post traumatic, I am certain that they would be met with several raised eyebrows. Most people are familiar with the term post-traumatic stress, as it is connected to the experience of Vietnam war veterans or victims of abuse. However, it is an experience that any individual may encounter when faced with a traumatizing situation, either real or imagined. For many parents, colic is one of those situations.

Research has confirmed that all individuals, not just parents, clearly have an unpleasant experience upon hearing an infant cry. Infants initially develop three distinct types of cries: (1) a basic hunger cry, (2) an anger cry, and (3) a pain cry. By two weeks to two months of age, they also develop a fussy cry. Responses to these cries are very distinct. Individuals hearing an infant cry will likely experience changes in heart rate and skin conductance.

Out of all the cries, the pain cry produces the strongest response. Interestingly, this response is not only physical, it is emotional as well. This is particularly true for mothers. Mothers often feel intense anxiety and worry when hearing their infant cry out in pain or what seemingly is pain. Parents of colicky infants often believe that their infant is in pain. Imagine the responses of the parents who are subjected to their colicky infant's cries on a day-to-day basis.

Jason and I became hypervigilant to sounds that would awaken Tyler or set him off in some way. For example, I remember when Tyler was about ten days old, standing in the kitchen with visitors. Tyler was taking a nap in my colleague's arms. She held him like a football. She was at ease with him. Jason and I were envious. Our visitors were chatting away about how wonderful it must feel to have a new precious baby in our lives. We saw Tyler squirm in my colleague's arms and heard him make some noise. Jason and I completely froze. Our guests saw our bodies tense and our faces turn white. They apparently did not notice the baby's movements and were alarmed by our sudden change in behavior. Jason said, "Nobody move." One guest asked jokingly if we were having an earthquake. Jason and I laughed. It was our first realization of how traumatized we were by Tyler's colic. We savored every moment that was peaceful in our home and didn't want anything to disturb it.

When individuals are feeling traumatized, it is often as if they are in a trancelike state. They are aware of the things around them, but their reaction to these things is either hypervigilant or avoidant. Irritability, paranoia, and a cynical, self-defeating attitude may all come into play during this time of distress. Sometimes the best parents can do to get through the emotional storm of colic is to go on with their day no matter how hard their baby cries and no matter how embarrassed, frustrated, or upset they are. Remember, isolation is not healthy for you or your baby.

I remember a time when I was feeling incredibly isolated and needed some relief.

Tyler was eight days old. Jason was at work and my mother had just left for the airport. As her cab pulled away from our house (I was still under doctor's orders not to drive), I stood in front of my house with a pit in my stomach. It was the same feeling I had when I was eleven years old and my parents dropped me off at my first sleep-away camp. It occurred to me that I said the same thing to them then that I said to my mother at that moment. "I will be fine." Why was it so important to be so strong? Why not break down in tears and say, "I'm not fine, don't leave me, I'm scared, I don't know if I can do this by myself, please help me." I felt numb.

As I reentered the house, I heard him. Tyler had woken up and was crying again. I walked over to his crib and bent down to pick him up. This was the very first time I was alone with him since the two-hour spurt in the hospital when Jason went home to take a shower. I was still somewhat shaken by the emotions I was feeling. I tried to soothe Tyler by rocking him in my arms. There was music playing in the background. My mother had turned it on before she left. She was a strong believer that a house should be filled with music. I began to dance with Tyler. Each time I spun him around in my arms, he calmed down momentarily and then began to cry some more.

We danced for what seemed to feel like an eternity. Time does not go fast when you have a screaming infant in your arms. After about an hour of nonstop crying, Jason called. I was feeling terrible, both emotionally and physically. I was pushing myself to do things physically that

I probably should not have been doing because of my surgery, but what choice did I have? Tyler was not an easy baby. Things had to be done.

Jason asked me how the day was going. It had been a particularly difficult day with Tyler and it took every ounce of effort for me not to break down into tears upon hearing his question. Jason could hear Tyler screaming in the background and said, "I'll let you go." There was no way to have a conversation while Tyler was in that state, but I did not want to hang up the phone. I wanted to talk to my husband like a normal person. I wanted to talk to him like we used to.

Right when Jason hung up the phone I began to cry. Tyler was screaming louder than before and there was nothing I could do to stop it. I guess you could say I joined him. We cried together for at least twenty minutes before I gained control of myself. I had not showered in two days and was feeling awful. There was no time to shower, no time to brush my teeth, and no time to eat. My days were spent caring for my hysterical son.

I needed to get out of the house. I had terrible cabin fever. Jason would not be home for another few hours. I decided to go for a walk outside. There were plenty of distractions outside the house and I hoped that Tyler might enjoy the walk. I had no idea if this would help, but I was willing to try anything. This change helped for a few minutes when he immediately took notice of the changes around him, but then the crying began once again.

My neighbor was outside with her two children when I left my house. She came over to get her first view of Tyler. She said she wanted to come by, but the blinds were always drawn and she was afraid to disturb us. I explained that Tyler cried a lot and that this made it hard to venture outside of the house. I did not want to go into all of the details, but I had to tell her something, especially since Tyler was wailing as we were trying to talk.

I was growing more and more anxious by the minute because I could tell that Tyler was starting to escalate quickly. With urgency, I told her that I was going for a walk to try to soothe him and that I had to go. I apologized as I began walking away. I was both embarrassed and upset by Tyler's behavior. As I walked down the street, I passed several more neighbors. To avoid conversation and further embarrassment, I tried to keep my head down and sped up my pace. On occasion, I would look up and acknowledge a neighbor who was close in proximity.

I was struck by the variety of looks and comments that I received on my walk. It seemed that everyone had something to say either verbally or nonverbally about my screaming baby. This is definitely something every parent with a colicky infant should prepare themselves for. Colicky infants do not have what one would consider normal infant cries. Instead, they wail at the top of their lungs. It would be impossible for the neighbors not to take notice. In fact, one neighbor was mowing his lawn and looked up to see where the noise was coming from as we walked by. I thought at least from this neighbor I was safely out of earshot, but apparently I was not. Tyler's screams could even drown out the sound of a lawn mower.

Although somewhat embarrassing, I did not really have a problem with others paying such close attention to us. A screaming baby will always draw some attention by the nature of the behavior. What I had a problem with was the type of attention being paid by many of our neighbors. I understood the looks of curiosity. I also understood the looks of sympathy as we passed by. In fact, these I even somewhat appreciated. It was the critical looks of displeasure and even disgust that were surprising and hurtful to me. Therefore, it is this type of negative feedback that I think parents need to prepare themselves for most.

As you are reading this, you might be thinking that I was only imagining these looks and that my perception must have been distorted. This is a fair argument considering my current state of mind and increased insecurity. However, I believe my perception of the situation was very accurate. I did not perceive these looks from everyone, only from a select few. The looks of criticism and displeasure surprised me. I wanted to shout out "Hasn't anyone ever seen a crying baby before?" But I didn't. Instead, I kept my mouth shut and kept walking.

I am sure my body language and facial expression portrayed the way I was feeling because some individuals commented on the situation as I passed by. The comments were interesting. Some were helpful and validating, while others were unhelpful and hurtful. For example, one person said, "Oh, poor baby." This was somewhat sympathetic, but it left me wondering who the person was sympathizing with—Tyler or me?

Another person commented, "Someone's not happy." My thought: "Ya think so?" A third person stated, "He doesn't seem to be enjoying his walk; maybe you should try holding him." What did she know? It wasn't worth the effort and energy to try to explain something to a total stranger that they would inevitably not understand anyway. Still, as I was walking around the block I wondered, "Could these people do any better?" I had to remind myself that their comments were not necessarily statements about my parenting, but rather comments made by an outside observer who had no understanding of our current situation.

I decided to go home. As I approached the house, I saw my neighbor across the street playing with her two boys again. Would I ever get to the point where I could enjoy being with my son, the way she clearly was with hers? It felt like a million years away. I rushed into the house through the garage to avoid any additional conversation with her. I was feeling too deflated to talk about anything. As I closed the garage door I could see her smiling at me with a nod of under-standing. It was only months later that I found out she too had a col-icky infant and struggled with similar issues for four months.

Coping with the Long Days

One of the hardest parts of dealing with a chronic problem is that time seems to stand still when all you want is for time to go by faster. Parents often report that during the season of colic it is hard being at home because time cannot pass fast enough. Many of these people were either used to being out of the house for work every day or accomplishing many important tasks at home. This change in daily routine and lifestyle can quickly cause isolation and sadness.

One mother recalled that when she was working, her day went by very quickly. She would look at the clock, see that the day was over before she knew it, and realize it was time to go home. Having a col-icky infant was a very different lifestyle for her; one that she was not enjoying at all. She stated that while she was at home, she would watch time go by on the clock. The minutes and the hours passed very slowly with her crying infant in her arms, but she still watched. There was nothing else for her to do. She commented, "Waiting for my husband to come home from work was my greatest hope for feel-ings of happiness each day."

Many stay-at-home parents who have the support of a significant other look forward to the end of the day because it means that they will finally get some relief when their partner returns home. One woman stated, "By 2:00 p.m. on most days, I would start to see the light at the end of the tunnel. I knew it would only be three more hours until my husband was home." She said, "My thinking was that once he was home, he could give me some relief from my daughter." Her husband agreed, but added, "The problem was that even when I got home, there never seemed to be time for that rest and relief, no matter how much I helped out."

I remember when Jason would come home from work, as a dutiful, supportive, and loving husband, he would tell me to go into our room and lie down. He was more than willing to take over. The problem was that there was no way to rest and relax with a screaming infant in the house. Nothing could block the sound of Tyler's cries. I tried everything: TV, radio, shower, even Tyler's sound machine, but I could still hear him loud and clear. Unfortunately, not only did this lend itself to a very non-relaxing environment, but it led to feelings of discomfort and guilt on my part. How could I lie in bed (especially when it gave me no relief) when Jason was in the next room with Tyler who was in complete distress?

Many parents talk about being a team in raising their child. It is true that statistically men are much more willing to be involved in the raising of their children now than they ever were in the past. The desire for men to be a significant part of their child's life is frequently present in households all over the United States. When a family is dealing with a colicky infant, having the team-parenting approach is vital for each parent's mental and physical well-being. However, this fact does not make it any easier to employ.

Take for example the common family unit where the man continues to work while the woman stays home with the baby (at least during a maternity leave). The man works a long full day at the office in a stressful job and then has to come home to even more stress and strain. This stress and strain does not go away and often escalates during the witching hours of the night (right around the time the man sets foot in the door). It doesn't seem fair to the man.

The woman, on the other hand, has been dealing with the hectic world of new motherhood. If the colic is severe, she has been listening to her baby cry relentlessly throughout most of the day. In milder forms of colic she has busy caring for her infant and her home at the same time, which is a huge accomplishment in and of itself. The woman may feel jealous and resentful that her husband has had the opportunity to be out of the house all day and escape the chaos. After all, he did not have to listen to their baby cry all day long. This doesn't seem fair either.

In fact, they are both right. Colic is not fair to anyone involved. It is not fair to the baby, it is not fair to the parents, and it is not fair to siblings or anyone else living in the house. It is during these times that couples most often fantasize about their old life together. Coming home and spending quality time with one another is often nonexistent or at least significantly diminished. Having adult conversation with one another about their day, the family, upcoming events, or friends can become a distant memory. Making plans for the weekend often disappears at least for the time being. The realization that as couple you may not experience these luxuries again for many months to come can be traumatizing and upsetting as well.

Couples also complain that when a baby enters their life, there is much less time for intimacy, both physical and emotional. With a colicky infant in the home this time is decreased even more. One woman told me, "It has been weeks since my husband held me in his arms or kissed me the way a husband kisses a wife." She revealed that this was not because of a lack of desire, but because there simply was no time. For many people this sounds funny, but for the parents of a colicky infant it is strikingly true. As I mentioned earlier, even basic hygiene can be put on hold during the worst colicky times. These are things most people take for granted. Finding the time to take a shower, brush your teeth, and blow dry or comb your hair can be a challenge.

These challenges can lead to a feeling of *loss*. Loss of something important can feel traumatizing to an individual especially if this loss is unexpected and there is no time to prepare for it. It is hard for people to envision that parents with a newborn would experience a sense of loss. Most envision this time as the ultimate gain. Nonetheless, parents of colicky infants do experience a sense of loss on a variety of things. For example, they frequently experience the loss of intimacy, friendship, and togetherness with their partner.

The emotional response to this loss can be very similar to that of someone who is grieving the death of a loved one. I know this was true for me. At first, I was in the denial stage. I did not want to believe that Tyler was colicky. I wanted to believe that it was something else. If I accepted that my child was colicky, then it meant there was nothing I could do to help him. It also meant that we would be living this hell for another three months minimum. My denial led to repetitive visits to doctor's offices, specialists, and emergency rooms.

I entered the stage of *anger* next. I was angry about having a baby who was colicky. I was angry that I could not enjoy him the way that other parents were able to enjoy their newborns. I was angry at Jason for going to work every day and leaving me by myself. Why did he get to leave and escape the insanity? I resented him for it. I was angry that we had no family around to help us. I was angry at Tyler for crying all the time (as if he could have controlled this). I was even angry about being angry. It was a never-ending cycle.

I eventually moved from the stage of anger to the stage of *bargaining*. Praying to God was a common everyday occurrence in our household. I prayed out loud every time Tyler cried. I prayed by myself and I prayed with Tyler in my arms. I prayed for relief, answers, strength, help, support, faith, love, understanding, compassion, patience…you get the picture. It was one of the things that kept me sane. I told God that I would do anything to make Tyler's colic go away. Instead, it stayed longer with him than for the average infant.

After the bargaining stage, I entered the stage of *depression*. I began to feel hopeless about the situation. My futile attempts to console my baby led to feelings of helplessness. My inability to find a solution and fix the problem made me feel useless. There were many days that I felt like giving up. (For more information on depression see Chapter 3, "Diagnosing the Problem.")

The last stage that I entered was the *acceptance* stage. I began to accept the fact that Tyler had colic. I prepared myself for the long days and weeks ahead. I resigned myself to the fact that I would be spending these days trying to relieve my baby's distress and at the same time maintain my own emotional stability. This was different from what I had imagined motherhood to be. Therefore, it took some time for me to fully accept this circumstance.

Any change in our life circumstance can cause us to go through the grief process described above. Interestingly, individuals do not necessarily go through the five stages in order (denial, anger, bargaining, depression, and acceptance). Instead, individuals often experience the stages in a different sequence, skip a stage or go through two or three of the stages simultaneously.

In addition, individuals often go through the stages during different periods of time. For example, Jason and I were told by many sources that colic ends when the newborn turns three months old. We eventually accepted the fact that Tyler had colic and that it would last for this period of time. However, instead of three months, Tyler suffered from colic for six months. With the realization at three months that Tyler would be struggling with this problem for many more months to come, I entered the stage of anger once again. During my anger stage, I engaged in some bargaining. However, I skipped the stages of denial and depression and eventually went back to the stage of acceptance.

The intensity and duration of a grief reaction depends on how significant the loss is perceived to be. In other words, if you perceive your baby as having only a mild case of colic, you may proceed through the five stages more quickly. Conversely, if you perceive your baby's case of colic to be severe, then you may spend more time in the various stages of grief. This is true no matter how mild or severe the case of colic really is because your process is based on your perception and not on fact. Parents often contemplate if they have gained strength from their colic ordeal. Many believe they do, but the most important message to parents is that you will get through it.

In summary, coping with the long days of colic can be difficult for even the most patient individual. The varying emotions that arise for people challenged with this problem can be debilitating. They often feel traumatized and experience a variety of losses in their life ranging from simple to complex. Therefore, a full chapter has been designated to focus on the issues of loss (see Chapter 8, "Loss"). In addition, many factors can complicate an individual's ability to cope effectively with the problem of colic, such as sleep deprivation, feelings of guilt, and isolation.

Sleep Deprivation

Have you ever kept track of how many pieces of advice you received before having a baby that you simply disregarded or blew off without a second thought? Before Tyler was born, everyone told Jason and me, "Get as much sleep as possible now, because once the baby is born you will be exhausted and horribly sleep deprived." Our silent response, "Yeah, so what, how many times have we been sleep deprived in the past? We can handle it. We'll catch up." Our polite verbal response,

"Okay, we will. Thanks for the tip." This was one of those tips that I wished I paid more attention to. However, at the time, there were much bigger pressures and concerns for us. Sleep deprivation was not one of them. Little did we know how much this could affect our moods, attitude, patience, and overall well-being in the months to come.

When an individual is sleep deprived, he cannot function nearly as well as when he is fully rested. Despite this fact, the trend in our country over the last hundred years has been toward an increasingly sleep-deprived nation. In the early 1900s, the average person slept nine hours per night. In the 1970s, the total was between seven and eight hours per night. The *American Sleep Poll* in 2002 indicated that the average person gets just under seven (6.9) hours per night.

According to leading sleep specialists, sleep deprivation is a common condition that afflicts 47 million adults in America. Therefore, approximately 25 percent of the adults in our country are affected by this problem. There are several problems associated with sleep deprivation. First, sleep deprivation can interfere with memory. The brain's frontal cortex functions much more effectively when a person gets a proper amount of sleep. With insufficient sleep, the brain is less effective in accessing memory, solving problems, and even controlling speech.

Second, sleep deprivation clearly interferes with a person's energy level. Sleep-deprived individuals often complain of fatigue and/or lack of energy throughout the day. It is particularly difficult to function when you are tired, especially when you are responsible for caring for a colicky infant.

Third, sleep deprivation affects an individual's physical health. Sufficient sleep is necessary to maintain a healthy immune system. Individuals are much more likely to develop an illness when they are sleep deprived. An illness as simple as a cold or as devastating as a stomach flu can make caring for your colicky baby seem like an impossible feat. One of the most important ways to ensure proper health is proper sleep. Interestingly, even if you are a healthy individual, it is not uncommon to quickly show symptoms of early aging and early-stage diabetes when you are sleep deprived. This is true because a sleep-deprived body is less effective in metabolizing glucose. A decrease in glucose metabolism (often observed by up to 40 percent) commonly leads to symptoms that mimic early-stage diabetes. Fortunately, research shows that this problem is reversible. In other words, these physical reactions will disappear when the individual receives proper rest.

Fourth, sleep deprivation interferes with mental abilities. Activities that require sustained mental focus and effort, such as concentration, organization, problem solving, and decision making are much more difficult for the person who is sleep deprived. In addition, activities that require quick mental response, such as driving a car or operating heavy machinery, can become highly dangerous without proper rest due to a decrease in the person's reaction time.

Lastly, sleep deprivation affects emotions and mood. Frequently, sleep-deprived individuals become impatient, irritable, and short-tempered. Researchers acknowledge that insufficient sleep can lead to a loss of emotional control and even violence. Insufficient rest can also cause hallucinations. One mother once informed me that after several sleepless days and nights up with her colicky infant, she began seeing her dead mother in her kitchen telling her what to do for her baby. Although she clearly knew that she was imagining this because her mother passed away twenty years ago, it frightened her. She did joke that at least she received some helpful tips in her time of distress.

From an emotional standpoint, it is extremely common for sleep-deprived individuals to experience stress and anxiety. These levels both increase as a result of sleepiness, and for many this increase starts a vicious cycle. For example, when the individual who is sleep deprived experiences stress and anxiety, that stress and anxiety often makes it more difficult for them to sleep. This lack of sleep in turn leads to more sleep deprivation, and then more stress and anxiety, and so on and so on.

Insufficient sleep clearly affected my mood when dealing with Tyler's colic. I was less patient and more irritable and short-tempered. In addition, I experienced high anxiety and stress following the long, hard days of relentless crying. There were several times that I struggled to fall asleep at night. When I attempted to lie down and go to bed, I often found it difficult to turn my brain off. I remember many occasions when I was lying in bed wide awake, experiencing high levels of stress and anxiety. In an attempt to focus on anything other than my racing thoughts, I would watch the minutes go by on the clock next to my bed knowing full well that with every second that passed by I was losing precious sleep time.

Many parents have agreed with my frustration and have shared their own. One woman told me that she would lie in bed awake for hours telling herself to go to sleep. Her husband would reinforce this notion, explaining that this was her window to get some rest, but she couldn't. No matter what she tried, she would lie in bed awake at night reliving the trauma she experienced that day with her daughter, who had cried for eight consecutive hours. She stated, "I was painfully aware that with every minute that passed by while I lay awake in bed my life would be harder the next morning."

Sleep deprivation affects your overall well-being. It is important to take care of yourself and get the sleep that your mind and body needs. I realize this is easier said than done; however, finding a way to catch up on those lost hours is imperative for your health and the health of your baby, so make it a priority. Perhaps placing sleep high on your priority list seems unrealistic when faced with the challenges of a colicky infant. Would it help to know that total sleep deprivation can be fatal? Research conducted with lab rats show that when prohibited from resting, the rats died within two to three weeks.

The amount of sleep that each person requires varies. Most specialists agree that the majority of adults should spend between eight to nine hours asleep per night for their well-being. However, a small number of people function perfectly well on only three to four hours of sleep per night. In addition, the time a person spends asleep changes with age. For example, infants require much more sleep than adults. As they grow, their sleep needs change. Although different people require different amounts of sleep according to their different needs, the following is a general outline to follow.

0 to 2 years: 13 to 17 hours per day
2 to 5 years: 11 to 13 hours per day
6 to 9 years: 10 to 11 hours per day
10 to 18 years: 8 to 10 hours per day
Over 18 years: 6 to 8 hours per day

Feelings of Guilt

For months before the baby was born, people told Jason and me that the easiest time (and one of the most pleasurable) with a newborn is when they are under three months old because all they do is eat and sleep. We were told that you could go out to dinners with the newborn and over to friends' houses. I often saw people at the mall or at church or at the gym with their infants. Their infants were well behaved and peaceful. Over and over again, I would hear people say what a wonderful time it was to enjoy the sweet innocence and beauty of a newborn and to bond with them in those first few months of life. Jason and I had no idea what they were talking about. To this day, I have no understanding of that peaceful experience. Our experience with Tyler was the complete opposite. It was not wonderful, it was not bonding (with the exception of breast-feeding), and it was not peaceful or joyous. It was hard, miserable, and frustrating to no end.

Parents of colicky infants experience many emotions. One important emotion that has only briefly been touched upon but needs further investigation is guilt. When parents are feeling overwhelmed and faced with insecurities about their ability to parent, the thoughts that result can cause great amounts of guilt.

Earlier I mentioned that many parents struggle with the inconsolable nature of their baby's cries and in turn feel helpless and hopeless about their situation. These feelings can become so strong that the fact that they have a living, breathing newborn baby does not stop them from wondering if they made a mistake. One husband disclosed, "The fact that we often wondered if we made the right decision to have children at all is too painful to even think about, not to mention talk about with others."

When parents are having thoughts that are causing them guilty feelings, letters, endorsements, and constant well wishes from others do not help. In fact, they often lead to an increase in shameful thoughts and feelings among parents with a colicky infant. One woman states, "Most of the letters we received when our baby was firstborn talked about having a 'bundle of joy' and it being 'the most precious time of our lives' to 'cherish forever.'" Her husband added, "These phrases were foreign to us. We kept wondering what bundle of joy? What precious time? Why in the world would we want to cherish these moments forever?"

Obtaining validation that your experience is different from those who do not have a colicky infant is important. This validation can come in many different forms. It can be as simple as your partner confirming this point and sharing thoughts and feelings that they have similarly been experiencing. It may come from other parents who have a colicky infant and understand what it is like to suffer from this problem. It may also come from a parent who does not have a colicky infant but realizes the specific challenges your family is facing. In any case, receiving this validation can help diminish the feelings of shame and guilt that frequently develop.

I remember one time that I received this validation. I was speaking to my aunt months after Tyler was born. As I was sharing with her our experience with colic she commented that what we went through was "inhumane." The word startled me at first. It seemed so severe, so daunting. But she was right. It was inhumane. I have since used this word to describe the enormity of what we were feeling and experiencing to others, because the word felt so fitting. There are few words to describe the painful and emotional process that parents go through when experiencing a colicky infant.

Isolation

Isolation is common among parents with a colicky infant. Any person who has ever cared for a newborn knows that it is hard to venture out of the house with a baby. After all, even the most well behaved baby needs a well packed diaper bag filled with items such as diapers, wipes, ointment, burp cloth, bottles, formula, tissues, toys, and a change of clothes (to name just a few). This does not include the blanket, stroller, sun hat, and pacifier that simply cannot be left behind. Now imagine taking on this endeavor with an infant who is not happy and calm, but instead screaming and miserable. It would be a miracle if the parent ever got out of the house. The embarrassment alone keeps many parents locked in their homes with the windows and blinds shut to ward off even the nicest of neighbors.

When I was at home with Tyler on maternity leave, I felt as if I had no life; I felt utterly alone. In reality, I was alone with him most of the time. Some days were worse than others, but overall, my time with my son in the several months of his life felt like a living hell. Is this how a mother would describe the first few months with her newborn? I felt like my life was falling apart. I had no time to shower or brush my teeth. I had little time to do laundry. I did not cook or clean. I barely ate. I lost almost all of my pregnancy weight in the first five weeks after Tyler was born. I was embarrassed by his constant screams. In addition, as exemplified earlier in the chapter, if I tried to venture out of the house, people stared. They wondered why I could not better care for my baby. I grew accustomed to the looks I got. I am sure I was a sight to behold.

There was one particular time that I will never be able to erase from my memory. Later Jason and I would laugh about it, but at the time I think he thought I was as close as I would ever come to being suicidal. The night before had been a longer, harder night than usual with much less relief. Tyler did not sleep more than a few hours that night and I was up most of the time trying to find new ways to appease him. Unfortunately, that morning he was crying louder than usual and was less distractible. I was becoming more impatient with him and found myself to be less distractible as well. All I heard was his relentless cries echoing through the house.

Jason had called in the late morning and could hear how upset Tyler was over the phone. Jason thought for sure things would relent a little bit following such a difficult night. However, nothing had changed. Jason asked me if I was okay and I flatly replied no. He told me to "hang in there" and I became infuriated. Who the hell was he to sit at his nice desk in his nice office at his nice work away from all of the screaming and tell me to "hang in there"? I hung up the phone. I couldn't speak to him. I was too angry.

A few minutes later I heard the phone ring and knew it was him. I still did not want to talk to him so I didn't answer. For the next hour, the phone rang sporadically. Jason was trying desperately to reach me. When he could not reach me via our home phone number, he tried my cellular phone. Both lines were ringing almost simultaneously for the next thirty minutes.

I knew Jason was worried. Maybe it was cruel, but I didn't care. I didn't want to talk to him or anybody else. I was beginning to hate my life. I finally got the strength and time (remember with a colicky infant it is hard to find the time to do anything—including answering the telephone) to check the messages. Jason had left three messages on our home phone and two on my cell phone. Still, I was not ready to call him back. I was angry and resentful and exhausted.

I finally got Tyler to sleep and was looking forward to taking a nap when the phone rang again. I had forgotten to move it away from the bassinet and it woke Tyler up from his five-minute nap. I was furious. Mostly I was angry with myself for my stupidity and oversight. I could not afford to make these types of mistakes with a colicky infant at home. Most mothers would have soothed their infants right back to sleep, but this never happened with Tyler. He was awake and probably would be for several more hours.

I picked up the phone and it was Jason. He was angry that I had not returned his calls. He was extremely worried about me and Tyler. After listening to his lecture, which was almost inaudible over Tyler's screams, I tried to speak, but couldn't. I burst into tears before I could respond. I couldn't stop crying. Jason kept asking what was wrong, but I could not respond with words. I could only cry.

Finally, I mustered up enough strength to tell him, "I have to get out of the house because I feel like I am going crazy." I told him I would call him later, and I hung up the phone once again. With bloodshot eyes, uncombed hair, unbrushed teeth, and no shower, I ventured out of the house with Tyler to go on a walk. I had not been outside in a few days. We were still in the middle of a massive heat wave. Temperatures were around 105 degrees. I felt gross, but it was nice to be in the fresh air.

As I walked down the street, I noticed that nobody was outside and the neighborhood was particularly quiet (probably because of the heat). I felt like I was in a daze. It felt surreal. The only sounds that I heard were the sounds of Tyler screaming in the baby carriage. He was definitely not in a daze. At one point his screams grew louder and the unimaginable happened to make the day complete. I began leaking breast milk. It felt like water had been dumped down the front of my shirt. I was soaking wet. I looked down at my T-shirt and realized that I did not put my bra back on after nursing Tyler earlier. I was leaking milk everywhere. I had two large round wet circles outlining my breasts, which were highly visible on the front of my T-shirt.

As I walked past a parked car on the street, I saw my reflection in the window. I was a complete mess. I barely recognized myself. I could feel the tears starting to flow down my face again. I was glad nobody was around to watch my outpour of emotion. I knew I could not go home so I continued to walk around the block. As badly as I felt and as horrible as I looked, I knew I would feel worse going back to the house.

Just at that moment, I saw a black SUV driving toward me. It was the first sign of life in the neighborhood since I began my walk. As it got closer, I realized it was Jason. He stopped the car in the middle of street and jumped out with the motor still running. He asked if I was okay and began hugging me. I couldn't stop crying. I pulled away from him and said, "Look at me. I am a mess and I have no life." He kept reassuring me that things would be okay and would get better. I told him, "I can't do this anymore." I told him that I needed help.

Parents who feel alone and isolated can much more easily fall into a depression (see Chapter 2 for more details regarding depression). Therefore, it is important to recognize the isolation that you are experiencing and then find some relief from it. At the end of this chapter you will see tips on how to take care of the caretaker. Many of these tips include ways to avoid isolation and gain some support.

Stick with What Works

Unfortunately, for colicky infants, many of the strategies commonly utilized by parents only provide temporary relief. Furthermore, this relief is usually due to the strategy creating a distraction and not to the strategy itself. Recognition of this fact has led several parents to create things in their environment that can provide their infant with less distress. For example, Jason and I quickly realized that we might be able to use Tyler's intense awareness of the stimuli around him as a way to help soothe him. We reviewed what had been helpful to him so far (even if it was only temporary). We knew that sucking (breastfeeding) helped to soothe Tyler. We also knew that movement was helpful for him. Jason and I had heard about baby swings and seats that vibrate and decided to give these a try. The vibrating baby seat (which our friends swore was a saving grace with their infant) entertained Tyler for a little while, but did not do the trick. We did not own a baby swing and were becoming somewhat tired of buying baby gear that did not seem to work. Therefore, we decided to first try out our own makeshift baby swing.

That night Jason swung Tyler from side to side in his arms. His arms became the swing's seat as his body moved back and forth. Tyler seemed to enjoy this. He stopped crying instantly. This movement became hard for Jason, so he changed it around by bending forward and then back to provide a swinging motion. This provided Tyler with the same relief, but began to wreak havoc on Jason's back. Therefore, Jason changed the motion yet again and began doing deep knee bends with Tyler in his arms. Again, Tyler reacted in the same way—with relief. I sat nearby watching Jason in awe. He actually found something that worked really well. Jack Lalanne look out! Jason was not only finding ways to soothe his colicky infant, he was creating a world-class workout regimen at the same time.

This strategy worked for us, so we kept using it. Parents become creative during a time of crisis. You probably have some strategies that you have created on your own that work well for your child. Remember, what works for one parent and baby may not work for another. Therefore, whatever works for you, stick with it.

Many parents start with one strategy and then adjust or transform it into another one. Finding relief is a work in progress. For example, I was happy to find an additional technique similar to the one mentioned above that, although strenuous, was not as difficult to maneuver. I came across it almost spontaneously. One day when Tyler was in his car seat crying, I began to swing him back and forth (front to back, not side to side). Interestingly, this seemed to calm him even more instantly than the other ways of swinging him. When I stopped the swinging, the crying began again almost on cue. I played around with this idea a few times and noticed a distinct pattern. The swinging in the car seat was actually better than the other techniques. I think it had something to do with the fact that it provided a larger, steadier swinging motion.

Jason and I tried variations of the car seat swing. For example, we tried to swing him from left to right instead of from forward to back and this did not work at all. We tried to rock him in his car seat in a slower motion, which also did not work at all. We even tried to swing less high and furiously off the ground, but found this also seemed to be less successful. Unlike the physical body maneuvers that worked equally well, the car seat swing only worked well one way (forward to back). The biggest trouble we could foresee with this new invention was that it would take more strength and effort to execute. The infant car seat did not weigh much, but it did weigh more than Tyler alone.

We adjusted our technique by finding ways to use different muscles to protect our back and shoulders from too much exertion and strain. For example, sometimes we swung the car seat in front of us using our right hand, and sometimes we swung it in front of us using our left hand. Sometimes we swung the car seat using both of our hands between our legs while our knees were bent, and sometimes we bent forward to ease our back by leaning against a chair for support. In any case, Jason and I took turns because this constant motion was incredibly tiring.

During the next few days, we found ourselves swinging Tyler in his car seat all the time. When he was not in his car seat, we were doing the deep knee bends that he liked so much. It was the only way that we were able to get some peace and we were grateful. We were able to eat in peace with one of us swinging Tyler while the other had a meal. We were able to watch a television show or listen to some music as long as Tyler was being swung. In a strange sort of way, it felt like some normalcy was returning to our lives. However, after several days of this trick working beautifully, we decided there had to be an easier way. We remembered that a friend gave us an old hand-me-down swing set, which might provide Tyler with the same relief and give us a break from the manual labor. We put it together and tried it out. Unfortunately, Tyler did not like it. In fact, it had the opposite effect. Tyler cried more in it than out of it. It was as if he was saying, "Why are you changing things around on me? The other way was working just fine."

We tried three different versions of store-bought baby swings. Unfortunately, none of them seemed to cut it either. Tyler was either used to the way we were swinging him or spoiled by the attention of the "mom/dad swing." In addition, none of the store-bought swings provided him with the long swinging motion that he seemed to need in order to feel soothed. Manufacturers did not produce a swing that went as high as we needed to swing Tyler. I am sure that they couldn't for safety reasons. Jason and I always buckled Tyler into his car seat and made sure his neck supporter was in place before swinging him. We certainly did not want to have any accidents in the process of trying to relieve his discomfort. If parents attempt to utilize this strategy, they should be very conscientious about safety. Even though the safety belt should always be in place before swinging the infant in the car seat, the swing should never be high enough to cause the infant to fall out if he was not wearing it.

CHAPTER REVIEW

Preparation

* Know what to expect and prepare for the unexpected.
* Setting up some sort of schedule or daily routine can be extremely helpful when dealing with the inconsistent world of colic.
* Recognize that if your infant is severely colicky, he may not be easily placed on a schedule. In other words, be prepared to go with the flow.

Psychological Ramifications to the Parent

* The constant cries of colic are not only unpleasant, they can be traumatic.
* Research shows that all individuals, not just parents, clearly have an unpleasant experience upon hearing an infant cry.
* Parents often feel intense anxiety and worry when hearing their infant cry out in pain or what seems to be pain.
* Parents often become hypervigilant to sounds that could trigger a colic episode.
* When individuals are feeling traumatized by colic, they are often in a trancelike state.
* In this trancelike state, they are aware of the things around them, but their reaction to these things is either hypervigilant or avoidant.
* Irritability, paranoia, and a cynical, self-defeating attitude may all come into play during this time of distress.

* Sometimes the best parents can do to get through the emotional storm of colic is to go on with their day, no matter how hard their baby cries and no matter how embarrassed, frustrated, or upset they are.
* Isolation and ways to get some relief.
* Prepare for the unexpected and often negative reactions of others when they observe your infant crying inconsolably.

Coping with the Long Days

* One of the hardest parts of dealing with a chronic problem is that time seems to stand still when all you want is for time to go by faster.
* Parents often report that during the time of colic it is hard being at home because time does not pass fast enough.
* Many parents look forward to the end of the day because it means that they will finally get some relief when their significant other returns home.
* When a family is dealing with a colicky infant, having the team-parenting approach is vital for each parent's mental and physical well-being.
* Statistically, men are much more willing to be involved in the raising of their children now than they ever were in the past.
* Obstacles commonly faced when trying to employ the team-parenting approach.
* Colic is not fair to anyone involved. It is not fair to the baby, it is not fair to the parents, and it is not fair to siblings or anyone else living in the house.
* As a couple you may not experience luxuries such as adult conversation or making plans for the weekend for many months to come. This can be traumatizing and upsetting.

* Couples complain that when a baby enters their life, there is much less time for both physical and emotional intimacy.
* The challenges of colic can lead to a feeling of loss.
* The emotional response to loss can be very similar to someone who is grieving the death of a loved one.

Sleep Deprivation

* When an individual is sleep deprived, he cannot function nearly as well as when he is fully rested.
* Despite this fact, the trend in our country over the last hundred years has been toward an increasingly sleep-deprived nation.
* Sleep deprivation is a common condition that afflicts 47 million adults in America (approximately 25 percent).
* There are several problems associated with sleep deprivation, such as a disturbance in memory, energy level, physical health, mental abilities, emotions, and mood.
* The amount of sleep that each person requires varies. However, the majority of adults require eight to nine hours of sleep per night for their well-being.

Guilt

* When parents are feeling overwhelmed and faced with insecurities about their ability to parent, the thoughts that result can cause great amounts of guilt.
* When a parent is experiencing guilt, letters, endorsements, and constant well wishes from others do not tend to help. Instead, they tend to increase these feelings and cause the parent greater distress.

* Obtaining validation that your experience is different from those who do not have a colicky infant can help diminish feelings of shame and guilt.

Isolation

* Isolation is common among parents with a colicky infant.
* Any person who has ever cared for a newborn knows that it is hard to venture out of the house with a baby. This is even more difficult with a colicky infant.
* The embarrassment alone keeps many parents isolated in their homes.

Stick with What Works

* Unfortunately for colicky infants, many of the strategies commonly utilized by parents only provide temporary relief.
* Use the colicky infant's intense awareness of stimuli to help soothe him.
* Examples of strategies attempted by parents.

Chapter 7

Taking Care of the Caretaker

Background

The stress that can develop from being a new parent is often very difficult to manage. New parents are often so focused on caring for their newborn that they forget to take care of themselves. This is even more true for the parents of a colicky infant. As discussed in previous chapters, parents who care for a colicky infant often have no time to attend to their most basic needs, such as hygiene, proper nutrition, and adequate rest and/or sleep. However, if left unattended, this personal neglect can eventually affect the caregiver's physical and mental well-being, which in turn can then affect the newborn.

For example, many parents have told me that when they do not get enough sleep, it is much harder for them to be patient with their children. Recently, one parent commented, "When I am sleep deprived, which is all the time with a colicky infant, I am more irritable and easily frustrated with my baby as well as with the rest of my family." Another parent stated, "It is hard for me to be my usual happy and energetic self when I cannot even find the time to eat and take a shower."

Clearly it is not always easy to take care of yourself when in the midst of caring for and managing a newborn. The newborn almost always comes first. In part, this is illustrative of being a good parent. Placing your child's needs over the needs of yourself certainly is not a bad thing, however, it can become detrimental when the caretaker does not even put herself second. Therefore, a psychological perspective on infant crying—including ways to cope with this intense outburst of emotion and some specific ideas for ways that the caregiver can take care of herself in the process—are presented below.

A Psychological Perspective

I have learned through my many years of practice that two things cause great discomfort in most adults: prolonged silences and outbursts of emotion. Recently, I provided an educational workshop for parents with difficult teenagers. I talked about the discomfort that people often have with prolonged silences. I role-modeled ways to communicate effectively with a difficult teen and purposely inserted some prolonged silences in the role play. In every circumstance where I held a silence, a parent interrupted me with a question or a comment within a ten-second period. Ten seconds of silence can feel like ten minutes.

Similarly, and perhaps more extremely, ten seconds of prolonged verbal distress can feel like ten hours. That is why the inconsolable, relentless crying that exemplifies colic can feel like a lifetime. In fact, this prolonged display of distressing emotion is unbearable for most individuals. There are many research studies that have specifically focused on the level of distress an individual can withstand. Results show that these levels are low unless some intervention is made to help the individual cope. These coping mechanisms may be positive or negative. For example, an individual may exercise, meditate, write, or paint as a means to cope constructively. An individual may also drink, self-medicate, self-harm, or abuse others as a way of coping, which clearly can be viewed as much more destructive.

If we apply these coping mechanisms to the specific situation of colic we might observe the following behaviors. First, it is not uncommon for caregivers to go out for prolonged walks with their colicky infant as a means of coping with the baby's relentless crying. A close friend whose firstborn was colicky stated, "I remember walking for hours when my son screamed. It was all I could do to keep myself sane." A patient once told me, "I lost all my pregnancy weight in the first three months because for hours I walked up and down the stairs in my house. It not only soothed my infant, but gave me some sanity!"

It is also not uncommon for caregivers to place their newborn somewhere safe and to meditate as a means to block out the uncontrolled crying. Sometimes individuals will include their newborn in their meditation process in an attempt to send "positive energy" to their infant in hopes of soothing him. For example, a woman once told me, "I used to put my baby in her playpen, turn on my music, and meditate next to her. I prayed to the gods to stop my baby's incessant crying." Even though she reported that this did not work completely, it provided some relief and "made us both feel better."

I strongly believe that if the caregiver is less anxious and distressed, then the infant will also be less anxious and distressed. This does not mean that colic is caused by anxious mothers. Instead, it indicates that there is a correlation or relationship between the two. As I discussed earlier in Chapter 1, "Theories of Colic," there is specific evidence that distressing emotions experienced by a caregiver can directly affect the infant. Taking care of yourself is highly important for the caregiver (see Chapter 3).

Another positive coping mechanism that is not uncommon for individuals with a colicky infant is to put the baby in his crib, shut the door, and escape to a part of the house where they can listen to music, take a shower, watch TV, write, or paint. One woman with a colicky infant once stated to me, "I would do anything I could to escape the constant noise. It made me feel like I was losing my mind." Another woman said, "If my baby was going to cry no matter what, then I might as well try to find some relief for myself by putting some normalcy back into my life."

Some caregivers under duress engage in potentially unhealthy and negative coping mechanisms when dealing with their colicky infant. For example, many parents have disclosed to me that they turned to alcohol or drugs to "take the edge off" when dealing with their difficult newborn. It is important to remember that although alcohol and some drugs (downers such as benzodiazepines, which provide a calming effect for the individual) may initially take the edge off, later these cause great repercussions. First, alcohol and the drugs described above are depressants. This means that they can potentially cause greater feelings of frustration, anger, sadness, helplessness, hopelessness, and worthlessness. For the caregiver who is already experiencing postpartum blues or, more severely, postpartum depression, alcohol and/or benzodiazepines can very easily and quickly add to this depression, making it more severe and less easily treatable.

In addition, impulsive acts are something to be watchful of, as this is not uncommon for parents with difficult children. Individuals with colicky infants often feel like they are at their wits' end. Listening to an infant cry for a prolonged period of time can feel unbearable. Often these feelings become so strong that the caregiver believes their only way to find relief is try to "force" the infant to stop crying. This attempt may occur through verbal or physical means. For example, a caregiver may yell and scream at the infant to stop crying—or more dangerously, shake, squeeze, or hit the baby.

Remember, crying is the infant's form of self-expression. The colicky infant is telling us something through his cries. Maybe the colicky infant is complaining to us about feeling overwhelmed, overstimulated, or overtired. Maybe the colicky infant is asking us to help soothe him. In either case, he is communicating with us about his situation. If we do not understand that his cries are his only current way of communicating with us, then we risk becoming frustrated, angry, and sometimes impulsive. Therefore, utilizing specific strategies to maintain both your emotional stability and physical well-being is highly important.

Specific Strategies

Exercise

Exercise is not only important for a person's physical well-being, but for their emotional well-being as well. In other words, exercise is good for the mind and body. Physically, it increases energy level, cardiovascular fitness, muscle tone, body temperature, and mental clarity. It decreases cholesterol levels, blood pressure, and the risk of heart attacks. In addition, it helps the person sleep better and maintain a healthy body weight.

Emotionally, exercise often helps to increase self-esteem and self-confidence. If the exercise includes a team activity, then it also provides a social outlet. This is particularly helpful for parents who feel isolated due to their baby's colic. In addition, exercise burns adrenaline, which decreases stress levels and promotes a more relaxed state of mind. Research shows that physical activity alters serotonin levels in the brain. Serotonin is one of the body's most important brain chemicals. It affects sleep and waking cycles, appetite, sex drive, and mood. Altered levels of this neurotransmitter cause an increase in feelings of emotional well-being.

If you have any physical limitations or concerns, consult with your doctor before engaging in physical exercise. This is particularly important if you have not exercised for a long period of time due to pregnancy or if you've had a C-section.

If you are someone who dreads exercise, try to choose a fun physical activity. There are many different types of exercise that you can choose from. For example, walk by yourself or with others, go for a jog, go on a hike, take a bike ride, attend a yoga class, attend an exercise class, or dance—to name just a few. Sometimes asking someone to join you as an exercise partner can help motivate you and provide you with a positive exercise experience.

Many doctors note that exercising two to five times per week for at least thirty minutes each time is an ideal amount of time to improve physical and emotional well-being. You might be surprised how easy it is to accomplish this task. For example, think about walking instead of taking your car to a nearby store or mailbox. One woman told me that she began walking to the grocery store each day, so that she not only received cardiovascular exercise but weight lifting from the grocery bags she carried home. Another woman commented that on her day off from her baby, she often played golf. She began walking the eighteen holes instead of using her golf cart. Do not be afraid to get creative.

Rest and Relaxation

Proper rest is vitally important for the caretaker. When people are sleep deprived, they cannot function as well and their mood is definitely affected. In addition, their tolerance for frustration and distress will greatly decrease. The detriments of sleep deprivation are discussed in detail in Chapter 6, "Living with a Nightmare." Therefore, I will simply reinforce here the need for a good night's sleep. Most doctors recommend that eight hours of sleep per night is ideal for both a person's physical and emotional well-being. Naps during the day can help. Training yourself to sleep when your baby sleeps especially during nap time is ideal. However, I recognize that this often difficult for parents with a colicky infant.

Most parents with a colicky infant believe that their baby's nap time is the only time they have to accomplish other tasks around the house. Although this may be true, try to think about the priority of sleep and not about what you think you probably should be doing. Obviously, this is not always possible. Just try to do your best. At minimum, finding some time in the day to relax and rejuvenate yourself is important.

Relaxation can take on many different forms. Some people enjoy relaxing in their home and some prefer seeking relaxing activities outside their home. If you are someone who prefers relaxing at home, think about taking a long, hot bubble bath with candles and aromatherapy; reading a magazine or a book; listening to soothing music; and/or drinking herbal tea, such as Celestial Seasons' "Stress Tamer." Be sure to turn off the telephone so your time to relax is not interrupted.

If you are more interested in relaxing outside of your home, think about getting a facial, manicure, or pedicure. To save money, find these products at a drug store and do it yourself under a tree in a park. Many parents treat themselves to a massage day at a spa. Contact local massage schools for discounted prices (often as low as $25/hour, including tip).

Some people engage in forms of personal expression as a way to relax and rejuvenate themselves. For example, it is common for people to write. I have found that journaling can be incredibly therapeutic for individuals who are struggling with an emotional circumstance. It can help them organize their thoughts and feelings, increase insight into their problems, and make realizations about their particular struggles. Journaling can be incredibly constructive for parents with colicky infants. Other forms of personal expression include dancing, singing, drawing, and painting. Again, it really does not matter what form of personal expression you choose to engage in, as long as it is safe and healthy and works for you. The key is for the activity to provide you with some rest and relaxation.

Other Social Outlets

Groups are not the only type of social outlets that a parent with a colicky infant can engage in. For example, many parents have talked about renting movies with their friends or going to the cinema on an outing with their baby. Most movie theaters now offer either an early morning show or a mid-morning show for mommies and newborns. In other words, these show times are specifically designated for parents and their infants. Therefore, you do not need to worry about finding a babysitter. In addition, the people who choose to attend these shows are prepared for disruptions and are accustomed to hearing infants cry. I recognize that attending a matinee would not be ideal if your baby is severely colicky and tends to cry relentlessly during this time frame. However, for those who have babies that do not, it can be a strong possibility.

For those of you who simply do not feel like you can leave your house due to the traumatic nature of your baby's colic, try visiting a live theater online, for example ComedySportz at www.national comedy.com or Children's Musical Theater at www.cmtsj.org

Child Care

Parents often become highly stressed and overwhelmed when caring for their colicky infant. Therefore, getting some relief from the infant's constant crying is important. However, even with help in the house, many parents struggle to find relief. For example, one woman shared that she hired a nanny for three hours per day so that she could catch up on sleep. Her infant cried throughout most of the evening hours. She said that while she was in her bedroom trying to sleep, she could hear everything that was going on in her home. She could tell when her daughter was being fed, changed, walked, sung to, etc. Although at some level this gave her some consolation that her baby was being cared for safely, she had difficulty achieving her ultimate goal, sleep.

After living with a colicky infant for a while, many parents become hypervigilant to the sounds and activities around them. Nonetheless, the benefits parents can receive from obtaining some sort of help with their colicky infant is not only physically positive, but emotionally positive as well. Sources may include, but are not limited to, family, friends, neighbors, religious organizations, daycare, nannies, students, and nurses. Before making a final decision on who will care for your newborn, it is highly recommended that you check the person's references, perform an observational interview, and establish a proper working relationship. In addition, setting up clear child care expectations by providing specific guidelines to follow will increase the success of a leave of absence from your child.

Finding child care is not easy. I encourage parents to talk to other parents, family members, friends, and neighbors about resources. Often receiving a personal reference from someone that you know can be less worrisome and more comfortable. However, it is important not to assume that a personal reference is always a safe and reliable referral. It is still important to follow the recommendations listed above. Most child care providers are required to be fingerprinted by law. This legislation is in place so that authorities have a record of individuals with a criminal history of abuse toward a child. Therefore, you may want to inquire with your child care provider if he or she has been fingerprinted.

Another resource for finding child care is through your local schools. You may want to contact either your local high schools or the colleges in your area to see if they offer courses in child development. If so, the teachers of these classes may be willing to inquire about student interest and advertise a potential position. In some cases, the teacher may also be willing to provide you with a student recommendation. Lastly, contacting child care placement agencies can provide you with a list of qualified child care providers. The largest downside about this resource is that it is often very costly.

Support Groups

One of the greatest ways for parents to gain support when they are in a difficult situation is in a support group. There are many different types of support groups. Like other things we have already talked about, it does not matter what type of group you choose to attend as long as it provides you with support. Therefore, if you are a parent who is interested in gaining some support investigate the various types of groups available to you. Some options are therapeutic groups, mothers' groups, and religious groups.

Therapeutic Groups

In my professional practice, I facilitate several therapeutic groups throughout the week. I am very aware of the benefits of group therapy. Gaining support from others who share similar circumstances can provide an individual with support, connectedness, hope, and insight. In addition, it can normalize a circumstance that feels completely abnormal. Many parents with a colicky infant feel isolated. Joining a support group is one way for them to gain a support system. The group may not only provide them with companionship, it may provide them with answers to their questions, diminish their concerns, and give them helpful tips during this very difficult time.

While I was in the midst of facing the unexpected challenges of colic, a support group was recommended by my lactation specialist. I liked the idea of joining a support group. I could not help but wonder how many other women were faced with colic and what they were doing about it. The prospect of meeting other women who were in my situation and having the opportunity to talk to them about their struggles immediately calmed my fears.

It is important to acknowledge that all therapy groups are different. Therefore, you should prepare yourself that the first one you seek out might not be the best one for you. It is important to choose a group that feels comfortable to you. I strongly believe that the key to success in therapy is finding a good fit between the patient and the therapist, or in the case of group, between the patient and the group as a whole. This is imperative for the group process to be beneficial to its members. Therefore, finding a support group for parents with colicky infants would be ideal; unfortunately, these can be difficult groups to find.

Most birthing hospitals offer support groups for new mothers in general, but don't often create and run a group specifically for mothers with colicky infants. In addition, it is rare to find support groups for new fathers. These groups are most commonly found when the father is either a single parent or a widower. In any case, the groups are usually free of charge when offered through a birthing hospital and encourage mothers to attend until their baby is approximately six months old.

I had the choice of going to two different groups since there were two different local birthing hospitals in my neighborhood. Both groups covered the same topics and had the same format. The only differences between the two were that one of the groups was much larger than the other and they were run by different leaders. I decided to try both groups out personally to see which was a better fit for me.

Initially, many individuals have some concerns about attending group therapy sessions especially if this is a new experience for them. For example, it is common for people to worry about things such as cost, benefit, stigma, and group cohesion. In the case of a mother with a colicky infant, mothers often have additional worries. This is particularly true if the group they are planning to attend is designed for new mothers in general and not specifically for the problem of colic.

Common concerns among these women are that their baby will cry hysterically throughout the entire group session, cause a disruption to the group process, and obligate them to leave. In addition, many have concerns about finding support and validation among parents who are not struggling with the same type of problem. Before entering my first group therapy session for new mothers I remember wondering how in the world I could have Tyler in group therapy with me when he cried all the time? I certainly did not want to disrupt the group process and knew I would inevitably leave if his cries were relentless. Truth be told, if Tyler had been crying before the group started, I probably would not have even gone inside.

If you are a mother who has these concerns or ones of a similar nature, remember that mothers who attend a new mother support group bring their babies with them. Therefore, they are used to hearing babies cry during the group's process. In addition, most of these groups are informal by nature. For example, during the group process, many mothers breast-feed their babies, play with them, or soothe them in some way if they are crying. These activities are all welcomed because they are all part of being a new mother and caring for an infant. However, if you feel like you need to leave because your colicky infant won't stop crying, you can do so without any repercussions. After all, the purpose of these groups is to provide all types of new mothers with a place to receive support. Therefore, if this goal is not being met for whatever reason, you are not obligated to stay.

I would like to take a moment to talk about the way in which parents often feel misunderstood when faced with the challenges of a colicky infant. I remember when Pat told me that I should attend the meeting and not worry about having a crying infant with me because the other women would be used to it. On one level she was absolutely right, but on another level I could not help but feel misunderstood. I did not have just a crying infant. I had a colicky infant. There is a very big difference between the two. I cannot tell you how many times Jason and I heard people say to us in their efforts to be supportive, "Call me if you are feeling overwhelmed; I can handle a crying baby." We rarely doubted that we could handle a crying baby too; it was the colic that presented the challenge.

Parents with a colicky infant have to deal with blood-curdling, hysterical screaming that, at its most extreme level, occurs every moment their baby is awake. As we have already discussed, it is different than ordinary infant crying, which is difficult to explain to others who have not experienced it. Many parents talk about how others—even close family and friends—do not fully understand the depths of their challenges unless they spend time with the colicky infant. Once that occurs, however, comments such as "I had no idea the crying was so bad," "How can you stand it? I would go crazy," or "Are you sure he is okay?" often emanate after only a few minutes of experiencing the colicky screams. These comments can be highly validating and indicate a greater level of understanding.

Be prepared that if you choose to attend a group that is focused on the support of new mothers in general rather than one that is specifically focused on colic, you may initially encounter some level of misunderstanding. In fact, you may need to be the spokesperson in the group for colic if nobody else is faced with this problem. Do not be afraid to voice the additional challenges that you encounter with a colicky infant. Other group members will voice their individual struggles as well. For example, you may encounter mothers in the group who may face unique challenges like handling triplets, caring for a disabled child, or being a single parent. Hopefully with time and support, all mothers will feel validated, supported, and understood.

I remember my very first group experience as if it was yesterday. Looking back on it is comical, but in the moment it was scary, embarrassing, and highly stressful. Tyler was nine weeks old. I arrived at the hospital and was happy that Tyler fell asleep in the car. I carried him into the group room in his car seat. The room was much larger than I had imagined. The group was held in one of the hospital's auditoriums. There was space for hundreds of people. I would estimate that thirty new mothers were in attendance, each with their newborns. Most gathered in the first few rows of seats and many mothers sat on the floor beneath the stage. Many of them brought blankets with them, which they laid down on the floor. They placed their newborns on top of these blankets and surrounded themselves with toys and bottles.

It was a very informal setting. I observed mothers playing, holding, singing, breast-feeding, etc., with their infants while the discussion group went on. The group members were diverse. There were women of all ages, races, and socioeconomic status. The one thing that everyone had in common was that they were all first-time mothers. I strategically placed myself in an aisle seat in the center of the auditorium. This was the perfect location for my comfort level. I was close enough to the front of the room to hear the group discussion, but far enough away for a fast and easy exit if Tyler woke up and began screaming.

The leader of the group began the discussion by asking everyone how their week had gone. Many women talked about their struggles with breast-feeding, mood swings, sleep deprivation, sex, weight gain, etc. I remember sitting there in a daze listening as the women talked about their various struggles, which, although very real for them, seemed so simplistic to me. I wished I had those problems instead of my own. Of course, I did not say a word about this to anyone in the group. I knew that would sound unsupportive, invalidating, and condescending. So I just sat there and listened.

At one point, I thought I might actually have something in common with a few women who began talking about their babies' struggles with gassiness. One woman had twin boys who were two months old. She said the boys were very uncomfortable after meals. She provided the group with a tip of how to relieve this discomfort. She stated that her pediatrician told her to get Mylicon drops, which helped with gas. She said it worked really well for her boys. She gave them the appropriate dose after every meal and it helped to expel their gas. Another woman agreed. She also had a baby who was uncomfortable after most meals until she was able to pass gas. This mother stated that she was using gripe water, which was helping her baby handle the abdominal distress she was under.

The first woman went on to say that she felt lucky to have tough boys who, even when clearly uncomfortable, did not cry. She had heard of babies who cried a lot with tummy troubles. I guess this was my opening to say something in the group, but I didn't. I could have inquired about the difference between Mylicon drops and gripe water, or I could have shared my experiences with Tyler's tummy trouble. However, I was still not sure how to explain what I was dealing with to people who were not experiencing it themselves. In retrospect, I guess I did not want it to sound like a superficial issue.

The group was ninety minutes in length. There was about fifteen minutes left when I saw a woman motion to the leader to look up in my direction. The woman had mumbled a comment of concern to the leader, which was not audible to my ears, that I assumed was about my well-being. I suppose she was concerned. My appearance, coupled with my lack of participation and isolation from the group, led to the leader's inquiry about who I was and how I was handling motherhood.

I had no choice now; I knew I would have to say something to the group. I started by introducing myself to the group and then introducing Tyler, who amazingly was still sleeping. The group members knew it was my first time there; however, I clarified this point anyway. I explained that my lactation specialist referred me to the group to gain some support from other new mothers. I told the group that I did not have family in the area and that my adjustment to motherhood had not been easy for me.

In an attempt to be nice, the leader commented that my son seemed to be the best behaved infant in the room. She said, "I have not heard a peep out of him the whole group session." I almost fell out of my chair upon hearing her comment. I never in a million years expected to hear something like that about Tyler—not now anyway, while he was still so colicky. I think all of the mothers in the room recognized my surprise, but nobody said a word. The silence led to a feeling of mild tension. Nobody knew what to say, including myself. Thankfully, the leader picked up on this awkwardness and quickly backpedaled. She said, "But you said motherhood has not been easy for you. Would you be willing to share your struggles with us? Maybe we can help."

At first, I wasn't quite sure how to respond. I was still shocked by her words. However, my shock was overridden with a sense of longing. I wanted to share my story with these women and gain some support. It was the whole reason I came in the first place. I just didn't know where to start. Also, I found myself holding on to the leaders' words. It was as if I was savoring them in an attempt to make them true. I was afraid that once I began telling the group members about my ordeal during the past two months, I would lose the title of having "the best behaved infant in the room" and it was nice to hear someone say something so wonderful about my son. I guess part of me did not want to ruin that.

After very little contemplation, I decided to tell the group my story. I proceeded to go through the long, tedious tale of Tyler's colic and the ways in which it has affected everyone in our household. I must have depicted a very real picture of what it is like to have a colicky infant because the group members seemed to be in absolute dismay upon hearing my description of the past months. You could hear a pin drop in the room as I talked about the eight-hour bouts of relentless screaming with no reprieve. I described the resulting feelings of hopelessness and helplessness experienced by me and my husband.

As I listened to myself speak, it occurred to me that although I felt like I had very little understanding of this problem with very few answers, I was beginning to sound like an expert on colic. I described to the group the trauma that resulted from being around a colicky infant. My husband and I were actually experiencing some signs and symptoms of post-traumatic stress disorder.

As discussed in a previous chapter, post-traumatic stress disorder is diagnosed when an individual has been exposed to a traumatic event in which the person's response involves intense fear, helplessness, or horror. The traumatic event must be persistently re-experienced in fantasy; there must be a persistent avoidance of stimuli associated with the traumatic event; and there must be persistent symptoms of increased arousal present in the individual following the traumatic event, such as hypervigilance, irritability, difficulty falling asleep, or difficulty concentrating.

Many parents experience these symptoms when they struggle with infant colic in their home. Sharing these experiences with others can be highly beneficial and lead to a decrease in symptomatology. Knowing this, I decided to talk about the devastating feelings that colic caused for Jason and me, including anger, resentment, sadness, fear, and disbelief. Perhaps most important, I tried to relay the message that the adjustment to motherhood was hard enough without having to cope with a colicky infant. I described to the group how the pressures, confusion, and uncertainty about how to handle the situation often left me feeling negative about myself. I concluded by describing in detail my personal experience with the negative thoughts I was having regarding my abilities as a parent.

Talking about your struggles and the challenges you and your family face each day with a colicky infant can be extremely therapeutic. Research shows that individuals who do not express their distressing thoughts and feelings often have heightened levels of stress. This increase in stress can lead to anxiety and/or symptoms of depression. Therefore, sharing these thoughts and feelings with other people (such as in a support group) can prove to be beneficial. However, be prepared that you may not get the response that you are looking for or hoping for from these people.

Upon the completion of my description of my ordeal to group members there was silence in the room. The silence was so thick that I was actually afraid that I might have traumatized some of the women simply by telling my story. Nobody in the room said a word, including the group leader. They all just sat there either looking at me or looking down at the floor. Some were distracted by their own infants, which seemed to be a nice diversion for them.

I could tell by the group members' expressions that they were surprised and sympathetic. However, their expressions also told a very different story. It was clear that none of these women had shared any of the same experiences that I had been talking about for the past fifteen minutes. Although sympathetic to my feelings, there was still a lack of full understanding. These group members were understandably unable to grasp fully the enormity of my situation because they had not experienced anything like it themselves. Although frustrating, I came to accept this fact.

The group leader was the one to finally break the silence. She reflected, "It seems like you are really going through a tough time." Several group members stated that the first few months are always the hardest and tried to provide support by telling me to "hang in there." Other members clearly did not know what to say so they simply commented that I should come to as many meetings as I could so that I would not be so isolated in my effort to handle my son.

I took this comment to heart. Upon hearing it, something very important occurred to me. I began to acknowledge that I could get support from others who were not in the same situation as I was. I don't know why I did not recognize this fact sooner. After all, this is the premise from which I work as a clinical psychologist. I have not personally experienced all of the things my patients have experienced, but that does not mean that I cannot help them and support them through their life struggles. It is so different when you are on the other side of things. It was both enlightening and educational for me to be in this situation and realize this.

Seasoned group therapists will attempt to provide all group members with some support and sense of belonging. This is true no matter what their individual struggles are, even if they are different from everyone else's. Providing a group member with a feeling of belonging is a key component in building trust, support, and cohesion. If the group member feels supported, she will be more likely to return to the group for future sessions. If she does not feel supported, she will be more likely to drop out of the group and remain isolated from others. Obviously, this would not be ideal for the person who is already feeling isolated and alone. Most of the time these attempts succeed and the person leaves the group session feeling positively about the group experience. However, this is not always the case. Some attempts may fail. Therefore, be prepared for this, especially if you are planning to join a group that is not familiar with colic. These failures are not necessarily the fault of the group leader or the group members. It is often simply an issue of a good fit.

You may need to educate the group on colic. If you are living through it and nobody else in the group is, you will become the group expert on relentless, inconsolable crying. One woman named Susie described her struggles in group therapy when attempting to educate the other group members about colic. Unfortunately, her group leader's attempts to provide her with a sense of belonging failed. Luckily, in the end she still gained support from group members and reaped the benefits of this therapy. She explained that her group leader attempted to dissipate her feelings of isolation by inquiring as to other group members' experiences with infant crying. The leader began by stating, "All babies get fussy, especially in the evening hours." She proceeded to speak about a "baby's fussy time," referring to this time as "the witching hours."

In a gracious attempt to gain some support for her, she asked the group, "How many of you have dealt with fussy infants like Susie has before?" Not a single person raised their hand. They all just sat there in silence. The only ones making noise were some of the newborns by their mothers' sides. Surprised, the group leader persisted in her questioning. She clearly wanted to make this woman feel better. Instead, she said, "Come on, ladies, nobody has experienced something like this before? We are talking about fussy babies here. Surely *someone* has experienced something similar."

The woman felt like screaming. She wanted to proclaim, "That is not what we are talking about at all. We are talking about *colicky* babies and there is a huge difference." However, she did not. Instead, she held her tongue and remained polite. She reminded herself that most people simply would never be able to grasp what it is like to have a colicky infant because they don't have one. This reminder made the process of being misunderstood much more bearable for her. She desperately wanted people to understand her experience so that she could get the validation and support she was looking for. Most parents with colicky infants feel this way. Fortunately, instead of this woman feeling sorry for herself, she began to feel relieved. She was able to take some pressure off herself and internalize the fact that having a colicky baby is not about something that she is doing wrong, but rather simply the way it is.

Only after several months of colic and many group sessions did I come to realize why wherever I went and whomever I spoke to about having a colicky infant, I was left feeling so isolated and alone. During that time, there were no people with colicky infants with whom to speak. I was not in a support group with other people who experienced this situation. They were all in "lock-down" mode in their homes. They rarely ventured outside of the house. Their window shades were drawn, their houses were dark, and they did not dare to put themselves in an embarrassing or anxiety-provoking situation in public.

In other words, the reason nobody in the group responded yes to the group leader's question of having a similar experience was because none of them ever had. The women who were struggling with colicky infants were not at that meeting. They were not attending any meetings. They were all at home—at least in the cases of more severe colic.

There were times I surprised myself that I attended group meetings and ventured out of the house. In fact, it was rare that I ever did. Group therapy sessions and doctor's appointments seemed to be my biggest outings in the first several months of Tyler's life.

I remember that first group session vividly. Just as I finished telling my story about my struggles with colic, Tyler woke up, almost as if on cue. He immediately began to cry in furious tones. His shrieking echoed throughout the auditorium. I stood up and said to the group members "Perfect timing." I could feel everyone's eyes on me. A little embarrassed, but somewhat glad that they got a chance to see what I was dealing with, I stated, "Some people like to make a grand entrance; we like to make a grand exit. See you all next week."

Gaining acceptance from others is vitally important to an individual's overall well-being. Therapeutic groups are a wonderful source of support. However, the group that you join does not necessarily need to be *therapeutic* in the formal sense of the word. I say this because not all groups are created for specific mental health issues, yet still provide some therapeutic value to members simply due to the nature of what the group represents. Groups are often created with the goal of building alliances, cohesion, and connectedness among members. Providing support and offering a sense of belonging can thus be found in groups that range in focus from a chess club to a battered women's support group. Therefore, as you search for a group that is right for you, remember that, to some degree, it really doesn't matter what the group's focus is as long as you find comfort from the people in it.

My goal in attending the new mother's support was two-fold. First, by attending I could gain some support from others even if there were no answers. Second, I would take myself out of isolation. Being in "lock-down" mode was definitely depressing and lonely. I knew group therapy could help me significantly with this. Following you will see ideas for groups other than therapeutic support groups that may provide you with some form of support and validation.

Mothers' Groups

There are a variety of mothers' groups located throughout the country. Some have a specific focus and some do not. Some are formally created and some are informally created. The ones that are formally formed by large organizations are either regionally or nationally known. For example, La Leche League is a worldwide organization that is dedicated to helping families positively experience breast-feeding. The ones that are informally formed are smaller in size and particular to a certain city. For example, it is common for mothers who meet under certain circumstances such as at the park or a play gym to form their own groups. In either case, most mothers' groups often join women with similarly aged children together to provide support and facilitate socialization.

Many of these groups stay connected as the children grow older. One woman with a son in college once told me that she is still friends with and frequently spends time with the women she met when her baby was three months old. Within these groups, members often share helpful tips with one another and are wonderful resources for a variety of parenthood issues. If you are interested in finding a local mothers' group, ask other mothers what type of groups they are in, inquire with your OB/GYN about her resources, and look in local community center or recreation department catalogs for mothers' groups. In addition, you can search online to find some options.

Religious Groups

Several religious organizations offer some sort of support to care-givers. Inquire about the type of support offered, which may include women's groups, mothers' groups, support groups, child care, Mommy and Me classes, etc. In addition, these groups often provide some form of daycare for children while parents are in attendance, thus making consistent participation in the group less stressful.

CHAPTER REVIEW

Background

* The stress that can develop from being a new parent is often very difficult to manage.
* New parents are often so focused on caring for their newborn that they forget to take care of themselves in the process.

A Psychological Perspective on Crying and How to Cope

* Two things cause great discomfort in most adults: prolonged silences and outbursts of emotion.
* The level of distress that an individual can withstand is low unless some intervention is made to help the individual cope.
* These coping mechanisms may be positive or negative.
* If we do not understand that a colicky infant's cries are his only current way of communicating with us, then we risk becoming frustrated, angry, and sometimes impulsive.

Specific Ideas

Exercise

* Exercise is good for the mind and body.
* If you have any physical limitations or concerns, consult your doctor before engaging in physical exercise.
* If you are someone who dreads exercise, try to choose a fun physical activity.
* Many doctors note that exercising two to five times per week for at least thirty minutes each time is an ideal amount of time to improve physical and emotional well-being.

Rest and Relaxation
* Eight hours of sleep is ideal and recommended by most doctors.
* Naps during the day can help.
* Ideas for relaxation both inside the home and outside the home.
* Personal forms of expression.

Other Social Outlets
* Ideas for other social outlets.

Child Care
* Getting some relief from the colicky infant's constant crying is important.
* Sources may include but are not limited to family, friends, neighbors, religious organizations, daycare, nannies, students, and nurses.
* Precautions to take before making a final decision on child care.

Support Groups

Therapeutic Groups
* Gaining therapeutic support from others who share similar circumstances can provide an individual with support, connectedness, hope, and insight.
* Group therapy can normalize a circumstance that feels completely abnormal.
* All therapy groups are different. Choose the best one for you.
* Initially, many individuals have some concerns about attending group therapy sessions.

* If you choose to attend a group that is focused on the support of new mothers in general rather than one that is specifically focused on colic, you may initially encounter some level of misunderstanding.
* Personal stories about group therapy.

Mothers' Groups

* There are a variety of mothers' groups located throughout the country.
* Some have a specific focus and some do not.
* Some are formally created and some are informally created.
* Many members of these groups stay connected as their children grow older.
* Resources as to where to find these groups are listed.

Religious Groups

* Several religious organizations offer some sort of support to caregivers.
* These groups often provide daycare.

Chapter 8

Loss

Description of Loss

Most parents who have a colicky infant not only experience a sense of being "locked-down" and "traumatized" while dealing with their colicky infant, they also experience a sense of loss. This is hard for most people to understand. They wonder how parents can feel loss when they are with their baby all the time. The loss can be described as a loss of time positively spent with your newborn. It can also be described as a loss of experiences to be shared with him or her.

The loss of time for many parents is profound. For example, one family disclosed to me that whenever they were with their baby, they constantly found themselves watching the clock, minute by minute, hour by hour, until the day drew to an end. Their reasons for paying such close attention to time were drastically different than for most parents. They watched time go by so that at the end of the day they could feel some relief. Relief that they got through one more *miserable* day. Relief that they were one day closer to their son being three months old and outgrowing this *terrible* time.

This couple kept telling themselves, "It will not be like this forever," even though it felt that way to them in the moment. They knew that with time, things would get better. Thus, they found themselves counting the days waiting for things to improve. Basically, they were wishing that time would go by more quickly. They actually wanted their son to grow up faster. Parents without a colicky infant would not customarily wish for this. Therefore, it is apparent once again that there is a huge difference in the experience of parenthood between parents with a colicky infant and those without.

I often hear parents talk about how fast time goes by when raising a child. They tell new parents to savor every moment because, "Before you know it, your baby will be all grown up." Many parents with a colicky infant have no concept of this idea. This is particularly true in the more severe cases of colic, when an infant cries sixteen hours a day every day for months at a time. These parents don't even contemplate the idea of wanting time to go slow—or even worse, to stand still—because for them, this time is not enjoyable. In their minds they have good reason for wanting time to move quickly. They want to start enjoying their time with their newborn. They clearly are not having the same experiences as most everyone else and they want to start having them.

This is true not only for parents with a colicky infant but also for others close to the family such as grandparents, godparents, siblings, cousins, and friends. All of these people may mourn the loss of positive, peaceful time spent with the newborn. For example, I felt absolutely terrible for my mother during her first visit with Tyler. I kept thinking about how miserable the whole experience must have been for her. She came all the way from New York to meet and visit with her first grandchild. Instead of wonderful, sweet memories of his first days of life being created, she was faced with a child who relentlessly screamed bloody murder and who caused pure exhaustion for all of those around him. She left having been invaluable to us but looking and feeling completely exhausted.

Most people cherish the moments that they spend with a newborn. They watch time go by with a sense of sadness because they recognize that they will never get that time back with their child. For parents with a colicky infant, not only do they frequently *not* want that time back, they don't want it when they have it. It is a terrible feeling of loss. This line of thinking is hard for most people to understand. In fact, I would bet that some of you reading this book are wondering how some parents could even think such things about the time spent with their child. If the circumstances were different for them and they had a colic-free baby, then the majority of them probably would never have such thoughts or wishes. After all, spending time with a newborn is a precious time of life and a significant life phase change for all family members involved. However, in the worst case scenario, parents are just trying to get through the storm of colic as best they can.

Since Jason and I shared similar thoughts, I can understand where these parents are coming from. In fact, many of the thoughts regarding wanting time to go by more quickly got me into trouble. These thoughts led to enormous feelings of guilt and insecurity during Tyler's first few months of life. It took me a very long time to come to terms with these feelings and an even longer time not to beat myself up for having them. At the time, I would tell myself that I had absolutely nothing to complain about. I told myself that I was lucky to have a healthy, beautiful baby boy. I reminded myself that there were many people who struggled to have children and many who were devastated to find out that they would never conceive. I reminded myself of all the children who were born disabled, deformed, unhealthy, or terminally ill, and the challenges that they and their parents would face in the long term. I reminded myself of all the parents who tragically lost a child in some twisted form of fate.

These reminders caused havoc in my brain. When all was said and done, I still felt sorry for myself and my circumstance and I was angry at myself for it. I chastised myself for being selfish. It seemed ridiculous to have these feelings when so many other people seemed to be suffering so much more. However, what I learned through my own process was that pain and suffering is relative. For me, having a colicky infant was a very real struggle and it needed to be validated as such. Therefore, I would like to send a message to all of my readers: *Remember that the people who are suffering from the trauma of having colicky infants are probably being much harder on themselves than anyone else could ever be.* They need understanding, compassion, and support, not criticism and blame. They probably give enough of the latter to themselves to last them a lifetime.

I do not believe that parents of colicky infants love their children any less than other parents. However, I do strongly believe that they become more resentful, angered, and frustrated by them. In addition, I think that parents fear that others will misunderstand the difference between the two, and in turn, either criticize or label them as being "bad parents." For this reason, I have chosen to speak openly about my true feelings. It is my hope that in doing so, I will be able to disperse the misunderstandings of others and, perhaps more important, decrease the parent's fear of being ostracized, criticized, and humiliated when speaking about having a colicky infant.

My loss of experiences with Tyler was profound. Jason and I never had the opportunity to do certain things with Tyler when he was an infant that other families could do with their non-colicky children.

These experiences ranged from small to large, simple to complex. I have spoken about many experiences already. However, I want to be more specific about some of our losses and the losses of other families.

When a baby is firstborn, many parents have high hopes of getting still photos, digital photos, and video footage of him to share with all of their friends and family out of town. It sounds simple enough to do, right? Wrong, at least not with a colicky infant. You might be wondering how long it takes to snap a picture here and there. The answer is too long if you have a colicky infant. For example, the only photos we have of Tyler in his first several weeks of life were taken in the hospital. Once we got home and the colic was in full force, not a single photo was taken by either Jason or me.

With a colicky infant, two hands are never enough. In fact, we proved that four hands could barely handle our son. To be honest, even with six or eight hands we struggled. Who was it that said it takes a whole community to raise a child? Even though the meaning of this statement probably has more to do with manners, morals, and values, it applied to us with our son. We could have used the help of the whole community. When a baby has severe colic there is very little availability to do anything else other than comfort him.

For many parents incentive plays a big part. If a baby is in constant distress any photos or video footage that is taken will only reveal his distress. Many parents indicate that their well-meaning family members who come to visit the baby naturally want to take photos of the precious newborn. However, the result is photos depicting an unhappy, screaming infant. My mother was able to find the time to take a few photos of Tyler during her initial trips out to visit us. In each of these photographs, Tyler was either screaming or frowning. The only times that he looked at all peaceful were in photos where he was sleeping.

Many parents do not welcome visitors during the time of colic. It is stressful and unpleasant for all those involved. Therefore, neighbors are shunned, friends are avoided, and family trips are delayed. In most cases, nothing is meant personally by these avoidances, it is just too hard and often embarrassing for the parents. Of course this is not the case for everyone. I was glad to have my mother be a part of this process because she could validate how incredibly difficult it really was. I remember her telling me that when she arrived home from her first trip out to visit, she pulled out the few photos she had taken, and everyone asked, "Why didn't you take more pictures?" Her response was, "There was no time."

To exemplify this point further, one of my favorite pictures of Tyler is one that Jason took when Tyler was in the midst of one of his colicky episodes. I am trying to soothe him by rocking him in my arms and singing to him while my mother is standing by my side feeding me a peanut butter and jelly sandwich. I just did not have enough hands to do everything.

Parents quickly learn how to prioritize their needs with their colicky baby. Even a person's most basic needs (like food) can be pushed aside as a priority. I have heard numerous stories about parents not finding the time to shower or brush their teeth until given a break at the end of the day when their spouse arrived home from work. Some parents noted that even then it was questionable as to whether personal hygiene was more important than sleep. Sleep frequently becomes a basic need that is at the very bottom of the totem pole, even though it needs to be a priority. I think this is because adequate sleep is not something many of these parents have any control over.

Another example of loss that is commonly experienced by parents takes place very soon after the baby is born. Similar to taking photos of a newborn, many parents plan on sending out a photo birth announcement shortly after their baby's birth. However, many have no time to put something like this together and no photo to attach. I was in this situation with Tyler. Luckily, when Tyler was a few weeks old, my in-laws were out for a visit. I am still grateful to this day that my mother-in-law took it upon herself to take some pictures while Tyler was sleeping. She put together a birth announcement for us. If she did not take the initiative to do so, I am certain none would have ever gone out. It just wasn't a priority for us. Photos and birth announcements may seem like small potatoes to some people. In the larger scheme of things, they were. However, sometimes it is the little things that add up and cause the greatest sense of loss.

The experiences lost by parents are numerous. One of the larger ones that parents often experience has to do with the social aspects of having and sharing the joy of a newborn with others. As discussed above, during the time of colic, families rarely have people over to their house. I know at our house our blinds were usually drawn and the lights were off or low. When people do come over, many parents have no idea how they will handle their distressed baby and be sociable at the same time. Obviously, this provides them with a lot of stress and strain. Therefore, the interactions that on other occasions would be described as pleasant and positive are often unpleasant and negative.

In addition, parents with colicky infants rarely leave their houses for a social outlet. Most do not attempt to go out to eat or to go over to someone else's house because they know how their baby will behave. Colic cries are often much more unbearable when out in public around other people. Most parents, particularly the ones who feel embarrassed and responsible for not being able to soothe their crying infant are not ready to exploit this fact in public. In addition, they are not ready or willing to put themselves in a position to share their insecurities and feelings of helplessness with others. Instead, they rationalize that any attempts at being social are futile and tell themselves, "We wouldn't enjoy ourselves or would end up leaving early anyway." Due to these thoughts and feelings, when invited somewhere, most of these parents learn quickly that the best choice is to respectfully decline.

People without colicky infants (under most circumstances) have the opposite experience. They can go to social gatherings with their newborns and actually enjoy their time out with friends. Going out with a newborn gives the parents an outlet and allows them to show off their newest addition to the family. Many parents look forward to it. When Tyler was much older, I began to notice how frequent these outings actually were (or maybe I just noticed more because we did not have this luxury earlier). There were many times before and after Tyler was born that Jason and I have been out to dinner or at a party where people were huddled around an infant and his proud parents. In these situations, the onlookers were in awe of how wonderfully sweet and cute the baby is.

I have seen infants at weddings, funerals, church gatherings, adult appointments, nail salons, hair salons, auto-body shops, supermarkets, the mall, etc. Taking Tyler to places like this was never an option for us. We would have been mortified to have a screaming baby with us at any of those places. Not only would this have caused us great embarrassment and anxiety, but we were not willing to allow such a disruption for the people around us. The babies we saw out in these places were all very well behaved. A well behaved baby is easy to "coo" with and to "ooh and ahh" over.

Jason and I skipped many events due to our dilemma. I know several couples with colicky infants do the same thing. Events become prioritized by parents with a colicky infant and are usually attended alone, baby-free. For example, parents will attend events that are due to necessity, commitment, and responsibility, but not the ones for fun, interest, or excitement. Interestingly, even in the case of the former events, attending such a function without your infant is not an easy task. Jason and I were seldom placed in this situation. However, it was still hard.

First, we were worried about how Tyler was behaving at home with a baby-sitter. Was the baby-sitter pulling her hair out? Could she stand the crying? Was Tyler in good hands with her or was he being abused in some way? No matter how well you interview a child care provider and no matter how many background checks you do, you are never 100 percent sure. All parents know what this feels like. However, it is even more worrisome with a colicky infant. It is not easy to take care of a well behaved, easy infant. It is unbelievably difficult to care for a colicky one. It takes someone with great stability, patience, and understanding.

Second, the few times we were away from Tyler to attend some sort of social event, everyone asked about him. Seeing all the other parents with their babies and children enjoying themselves was unsettling for us. It also seemed unbelievably unfair. It never ceased to amaze Jason and me that the average baby could be so docile and pleasant. It was such a foreign concept to us. I felt badly for Tyler and for us. Seeing other people with their infants was a reminder of how his constant distress affected our family and strained our relationship with one another.

I want to share a personal loss of experience I had. This loss was particularly meaningful and emotional for me. When I was pregnant with Tyler I was in the midst of finishing up my pre-doctoral internship hours and completing my doctoral dissertation for clinical psychology. When Tyler was four and a half months old, I attended my graduation ceremony. My family and Jason's family flew out for this special occasion. It was the first time that we were all together in a very long time and I was looking forward to sharing my accomplishment with the group.

While I was in my doctoral program, I had often envisioned my graduation day. Since I went to a small school, I knew it would be a very small ceremony in which I could make a speech and personally thank all of those individuals who had supported me in my endeavors. I did not have the opportunity to do this when I received my master's degree from Columbia University because the school was simply too large and thus did not allow for the same type of intimacy.

I worked hard to obtain my doctoral degree. I went to school full time and worked full time in order to pay my own tuition without having to take out student loans. I was proud of my achievements and wanted to celebrate them on my graduation day. I came up with a fun way to make the day even more memorable than I had originally envisioned. Since I had been pregnant with Tyler all during my final year in school, I decided to surprise my family and do something special to honor my newborn son on my graduation day. After all, Tyler was with me while I completed my graduation requirements. It almost felt as if he deserved to graduate along with me, so I bought him a cap and gown that matched mine. I had to have it altered, of course, to fit his cute little body and head (they don't make caps and gowns that small). I even ordered an extra tassel so that we would match exactly.

I couldn't wait for everyone to see him. I was excited to take some pictures of us together in our matching attire to add to my very small, but growing, collection of photos. I kept imagining what a great opportunity it would be to create this memory that would last a lifetime. I fantasized about sharing this photo with Tyler when he was older and telling the story of that perfect day. Unfortunately, this fantasy never came true. I guess I should have known better. It was never meant to be with a colicky infant.

Tyler was particularly colicky on the day of my graduation. During the two-hour drive to the location of the ceremony, Tyler slept most of the way. A good sign (so we thought). When we arrived he was hungry. After eating, I tried to put him into his cap and gown. He completely rejected the idea. He refused to be dressed by me or anyone else (and I think almost everyone tried). He kicked and squirmed so much that it was impossible to get his outfit on.

I had to get ready myself, so Jason took over and with some help from above, somehow miraculously got him into his outfit. When I came out to take some pictures with my family, I could see Tyler was screaming. He was incredibly hard to soothe that day. All of the tricks that we knew to calm him even temporarily for a quick photo shoot were not working. Jason and I were literally sweating from our efforts. The few photos that were taken of us in our matching outfits featured me half-smiling (trying to fake it) and Tyler screaming his head off. When all was said and done, we only got one out of thirty pictures that was half-decent. Tyler was crying in this photo, but his distress was less obvious in this one than in the others.

After our photo attempts, the graduation ceremony began. I knew it would be too much to ask of Tyler to behave throughout the whole ceremony. However, I was hoping for some good behavior at least during the time that I would give my speech. I planned on thanking my family and wanted everyone in attendance. Unfortunately, this did not happen. As I stood before the attendees, I realized that my mother-in-law was not in her seat. I realized she was probably taking her turn with Tyler, trying to settle him down. She was nowhere in sight. I was saddened by the fact that she would not hear the words I would bestow upon the people in front of me.

As I got halfway through my speech, I heard what sounded like Tyler's cries far off in the distance. As I glanced out the window, the cries became louder and that's when I saw her. My mother-in-law was sprinting across the open patio pushing the baby stroller in front of her with Tyler in it. She was determined to get to the other side where she would be out of earshot once again. The patio was located directly next to the room in which we were all gathered. Tyler was crying furiously and everyone could hear him. My mother-in-law was running so fast, she was only briefly visible. The cries became softer with the growing distance. I thought to myself, "That's my son," and resumed my speech. I later asked my family for confirmation if I simply thought those words or if I said them out loud.

My family and I have had some good laughs when reminiscing about that moment. Even at the time it was somewhat comical. I think the most interesting part of this day was that I was not angry, upset, or even surprised. Of course, I was frustrated with the lack of good photos and the absence of family during my speech, but that was to be expected. I think Jason and I became so accustomed to situations like this that it did not even faze us anymore. It was not until many months later when Tyler was well over a year old that I thought about it and my sadness crept in.

Unfortunately, the loss of experience did not end there. Later that night, Jason and I hosted a graduation party for myself at a local restaurant. All of my colleagues, friends, and family were in attendance. I was so excited to have everyone together in the same room. It would be the first time that my family would meet many of the people about whom I had spoken so highly.

Having everyone together was something that I had fantasized about for a very long time. Whenever family comes to visit, which unfortunately is not that often, they do not stay for long periods of time. This is one of the downfalls in having family members who live out of state. During their short visits it has been difficult to introduce them to all of the important people in my life. I thought this would be the perfect opportunity to do so.

In addition, Jason and I decided to bring Tyler with us to this event since many of the people in attendance wanted to meet him. I had been in "lock-down" mode for so long that even though Tyler was almost five months old, many of the people in attendance who were close to us still had not had the opportunity to meet him. I was worried that he would have a very hard time at the party. If the earlier part of the day was any indication of what that night would be like I knew we would be in trouble. However, we followed through with our original plan and Tyler attended the party with all of us that evening.

Jason and I were the first to arrive at the restaurant. My parents arrived shortly after. The rest of our family followed later. As the initial guests arrived, I introduced them to my parents and Tyler. However, approximately thirty minutes into the party, Tyler began to have a meltdown. Most of the guests had not arrived yet.

My father volunteered to swing Tyler in his car seat. We all hoped that this would calm him down. Unfortunately, Tyler was in rare form that night. He cried so loud and for so long that my father had to remove himself from the party area and move to the back of the restaurant where there were no signs of life. My father, like me, had the instinct and desire to avoid disturbing the people around him with a crying infant.

To make a long story short, Tyler did not relent in his cries for the rest of the night. My father was stuck in the back of the restaurant for hours swinging his grandson. I brought some people back to where he was stationed to meet him and to meet Tyler. However, since he was not located where the rest of the guests were gathering, nobody stayed for long. Some people were nice enough to ask if they could help. However, most did not. After all, who would want to hang out with a screaming baby when there was a party going on? My mother, Jason, and I checked in on him from time to time. Each time we did, he had told us to go back to the party and that he was doing just fine.

At one point during the party one of our guests arrived with her three-week-old newborn. It was her first time introducing her daughter to many of our mutual friends. I watched our guests surround the newborn infant. They took turns holding her and cooing with her. She was wide awake and perfectly behaved. She ate, slept, and was changed throughout the night without fussing once. It is amazing how babies can behave so differently from one another. This little newborn was being enjoyed by many, while my son was in the back of the building being enjoyed by no one—except maybe his grandfather, and even that would be questionable.

My father gave me a wonderful gift that night. He allowed me to find some peace and enjoyment in my own graduation party by taking charge of my colicky son. I thanked him dearly for that. However, with all of my appreciation, there is an overshadowing sadness. In essence, my father missed his daughter's graduation party. Even though he was there he was, ultimately, *not there.*

My parents ended up taking Tyler home early that night. It was not the party I had envisioned for them. I wanted them to meet and mingle with all of my colleagues and friends. I guess it was silly to think this could occur with a colicky infant in the room. Suffice it to say, the loss of experience had occurred once again.

Acceptance of Loss

The loss of experience that parents face with having a colicky infant is hard to overcome. However, it is what it is. You can either accept it and move forward or dwell on it and remain stuck in your negative emotions. Jason and I chose to accept it. We believed we had no choice. We couldn't change it and we did not want to let it get us down, so we chose to accept it. Coping with this loss is only part of coping with the greater issue of colic. With colic come these types of losses. Therefore, utilizing the same strategies already listed in Chapter 6, "Living with a Nightmare," and Chapter 7, "Taking Care of the Caretaker," will help.

Lack of Acceptance of Loss

It would be hard for parents with easy children to understand the tremendous stress and hardship that can be placed on a parent with a difficult child. Although there were many times that friends of mine who had easy children shared their struggles and then said, "I don't know how you managed. I thought I had it hard."

Being a new parent is hard enough. Being a new parent with a colicky infant can be devastating. As I mentioned earlier, there were times when I became so frustrated and exhausted dealing with Tyler that I actually understood how some parents could lose control and harm their child. I kept thanking God that I had the stability and resources available never to allow this to happen to my own child. Nonetheless, I had a better understanding of how this *could* occur. It is an uneasy feeling.

According to the National Child Abuse and Neglect Data System (NCANDS) there are over three million cases of child abuse reported nationally each year. Approximately 30 percent of these reports found at least one child to be the victim of child abuse. NCANDS cited that an estimated 896,000 children were determined to be victims of child abuse or neglect in 2002. In addition NCANDS estimated 1,400 children died from either abuse or neglect in 2002. That is 1.98 children per 100,000 children in our country. Children under one year of age accounted for 41 percent of these fatalities.

Many researchers and practitioners believe that child fatalities are underreported. It is believed that impulsive or accidental acts by a caregiver that result in death are often not investigated, and are therefore underreported. According to NCANDS, in 2002 one or both parents were involved in 79 percent of child abuse and neglect fatalities. More than one-third (38 percent) of child maltreatment fatalities were associated with neglect alone and more than one-quarter (30 percent) were associated with physical abuse alone. The remaining percentage indicated a combination of maltreatment leading to death.

These numbers are staggering, yet they are not highly publicized. It is only the few cases that are so horrific to catch the media's attention that make the news. For example, the mother who drove her car into a river drowning her four children, or the parent who suffocated her crying baby. Did these parents have difficult children with little or no resources to cope? Even if the answer is yes, this does not excuse their behavior. However, this information can give us some insight into why it occurred and that information can potentially help us prevent similar situations from occurring in the future with people who are in similar circumstances.

Suffice it to say, gaining knowledge and understanding from individuals who have dealt with colicky infants could diminish the devastation that the parents and their family members face on a day-to-day basis. Furthermore, gaining knowledge of how parents with colicky infants cope with the immense stress they are under could decrease the potential for abuse and infant death. Perhaps with this recognition parents with little resources could obtain the necessary tools to prevent isolation, despair, and trauma.

CHAPTER REVIEW

Description of Loss
* Loss of time positively spent with your newborn.
* Loss of experiences to be shared with him or her.

Acceptance of Loss
* Having a healthy outlook on the experience of loss.
* Mourning the loss.
* Moving forward.

Lack of Acceptance of Loss
* Unhealthy outlook on the experience of loss.
* Lack of acceptance can lead to instability and potential abuse of children.

Chapter 9

The Road Back

Eventually all children outgrow colic unless faced with unusual circumstances. As we have already discussed in previous chapters, if your baby cries more often around the time that he is eating or soon thereafter, his distress is most likely due to his immature digestive system. In this case, his crying bursts will most likely subside as his digestive system matures. Most parents with babies who fit this description report that when their baby is around three and a half months old (remember the digestive system is fully developed at one hundred days old), he stops crying. In fact, statements such as "it was like night and day" or "one day he just stopped crying" are commonly heard in this situation.

For many parents, the circumstance of their baby's colic is different. If you have a baby who is crying due to overstimulation in his environment and an inability to self-soothe then there is no biological indicator available to you that can estimate the termination of colic. Some infants may present colic for three months and some for six months. It depends on the given child. For example, it was not until Tyler turned six months old that Jason and I considered him colic-free. For us, things gradually got better between three months and six months of age. We had our good days and our bad days and, like other parents, managed to get through them. However, as we neared the six-month mark, unlike other parents, on our bad days, Jason and I were able to remind ourselves that it was nothing like it used to be when Tyler was first born. This comparison seemed to help us get through the tougher days with less stress and more ease.

Having a baby who does not cry relentlessly is a very different experience for parents. It is only at this time that you truly get to see your child's developing personality because for the first time it is not overshadowed by his colicky screams. When colic is gone, parents are soon able to communicate with their babies in ways that they never could have imagined possible only a few months earlier.

Dr. Karp writes, "Once the colicky baby stops crying, he becomes the happiest baby on the block." This was true in Tyler's case. When Tyler was three months old, Jason and I began to see visions of what would be in our future with him. He began to smile and coo with us in between his bouts of intense crying. Each time this occurred our hearts melted, and we were reminded of how lucky we were to have such a precious child. We realized that these glimmers of hope were gifts. Tyler was clearly becoming "the happiest baby on the block" and we were excited about the transformation.

Tyler is the type of child who lights up any room he is in. Maybe this is due to his outward appearance, maybe it is due to his personality, or maybe it is both. Tyler has white-blond hair and striking blue eyes that sparkle every time he smiles—and he is almost always smiling these days. It is as if he is making up for lost time. He's a charmer, incredibly outgoing and sociable. He likes being around people and interacting with them. Before he could crawl or walk, he engaged people with his gaze, smile, and laughter. Once he became mobile, he was eager to approach the closest person to show off his developmental achievements.

Tyler reached all of his developmental milestones early. He sturdily held his head up within weeks of his life. He sat up by himself at three months. He started crawling at six months. He started walking the day he turned ten months old. By the time he turned eighteen months of age, he was running, climbing, jumping, and swinging just like a three-year-old. His size and coordination helped him in this capacity. Tyler has always been off the charts for height and in the nintieth percentile for weight. He is a strong, sturdy boy.

Tyler's physical achievements, although impressive, came secondary to his verbal achievements. He said his first word (in addition to "mama" and "dada") at eight months of age and has not stopped talking since. By the time Tyler turned one, he had a one-hundred-word vocabulary. By the time he was eighteen months of age; he spoke full sentences and had a six-hundred-word vocabulary. Tyler is now two years old, and many of our friends with small children call him "the linguist." Everywhere we go, people comment on his advanced verbal skills. What I often wished for during his colicky episodes finally came true. Tyler, my baby, could talk.

Tyler's verbal achievements have been a godsend. It is so much easier to soothe a baby when you know what is bothering him. Yes, Tyler is still a hard to soothe baby; that I will admit. As happy as he is, we still have our struggles when he becomes frustrated, angry, or sad. His self-soothing techniques are improved, but not perfected. I hope this will improve more with time.

I think it is important to note that although Tyler's colic went away as we knew it eventually would, his temperament and personality has not changed. These are stable traits and I am glad. I didn't realize it at the time, but his sensitivity to stimuli now presents itself as an overall sensitivity to the world around him. He is thoughtful and caring and sensitive to others even at his young age. For example, if we are engaged in an activity that he is clearly enjoying, he will tell me how much one of his friends would like the activity and that we should ask him or her to join us the next time.

Tyler often wants others to have what he has, which is somewhat remarkable for a child in the midst of the terrible two's. I remember shopping at a local superstore with Tyler when he was twenty-three months old. He had found a new ball that he was particularly infatuated with. I told him I would buy it for him. As we began to walk toward the checkout counter to pay for the items in our cart, Tyler turned around and ran back toward the balls. I watched him as he picked up three additional balls and carried them toward me. I asked him to please put them back and told him that we were only buying one ball today. He looked me straight in the eye and said, "But Mommy, we have to buy these balls. Papi (Jason) and you need one too." I asked him who the third ball was for and he replied somewhat impatiently, "Mommy, it's for Brody" (Tyler's little brother, who was two weeks old).

Tyler's sensitivity to others' pain is also remarkable. He is very tuned-in to others' distress. I wonder if this comes from being so distressed himself in his earliest months of life. When a child is crying, he looks to Jason and me and says, "That kid is crying." He then says, "I'll help him," and proceeds to go over to the crying child to say, "It's okay. Don't cry," as he pats him on the back. He does this all the time with his baby brother, who is now four months old. He consoles him by stating, "Don't worry, Brody, its okay Tyler is here. Mommy is here. Papi is here. We'll take care of you."

Brody was born when Tyler was twenty-three months of age. They are almost exactly two years apart. Tyler's sensitivity and caring is apparent in his relationship with his brother. Although the transition of having to share attention was difficult for him at first, he clearly is excited about having a little brother. He often tells me, "When Brody gets bigger, he can play baseball with me and eat pancakes with me and go on the potty like me." Tyler enjoys showing his little brother how to do things and finds pleasure in making him smile and laugh.

I know that many of you who are reading this book are probably wondering if Brody was a colicky infant as well. Everyone we knew told us that after what we went through with Tyler, we were sure to have an "easy" second baby. Some people could not believe that we even contemplated having another child after the trauma that we experienced with our first. After all, remember what the research says about having a colicky infant. You are just as likely to have a colicky infant with your firstborn as you are with your second, third, or fourth. Therefore, Jason and I were prepared for the worst.

We always wanted to have more than one child and, after much contemplation, we decided to have another baby sooner rather than later. In all honesty, the decision stemmed from my fear that if we waited too long and things got to be easy with Tyler, I might change my mind. Even though Jason and I felt much more equipped to deal with a second colicky infant if that is what we were presented with, the thought of *having* to deal with this stress and strain lay heavy on our minds. Of course, there was the possibility that we would not have to cope with colic at all the second time around. It is true that all children are different. Even identical twins who come from the same gene pool have their differences in temperament and personality.

So, let me answer the burning question that so many people have asked after hearing our detailed story describing Tyler's colic. The burning question: Was Brody colicky too? The answer: It depends on who you ask.

For the first three weeks of Brody's life, we experienced a new phenomenon: peace and quiet with a newborn. Brody slept well and ate well and, most important, rarely cried in between. He developed a predictable pattern very quickly, which made life much less stressful and much more enjoyable. Jason and I were thrilled. We finally understood what so many other couples experienced with their newborns. Unfortunately, this experience was somewhat short-lived. When Brody was three and a half weeks old, he began to cry more often. He was fussy most of the time he was awake. Unlike Tyler, his cries were softer and therefore much more bearable. However, they were still very present in our home. Even so, I would not have considered them colicky cries because they were so much less severe than anything we had ever experienced with Tyler.

There were a few nights Jason and I worried that Brody was becoming colicky. I remember those nights well. On two separate occasions he cried relentlessly for several continuous hours. I remember on both of those nights exchanging glances with Jason wondering if this was the beginning of more colic behavior to come. One night I clearly stated to Jason, "I cannot do this again." I remember wondering, "Is this really happening to us a second time?"

Neither Jason nor I could figure out why Brody was unhappy during these times, although it seemed like gas was the main culprit. What was different from before was that this time we had the skills to successfully intervene. Jason and I quickly pulled out all of our old tricks to cope with the fussy times. For example, we found that the Mylicon drops (to help with gas) helped tremendously. We also began swinging Brody in his car seat just as we had with Tyler for all of those long hard months. I remember watching Jason go up to the attic to bring down "the car seat" that was so present in our lives only a few years earlier. I was hoping never to use that car seat again, but was happy we had kept it in storage just in case we needed it. Swinging Brody in this car seat, which was much more lightweight than his new one, helped immensely.

Jason and I employed the techniques listed in Chapter 6 whenever Brody became fussy to give him and us some relief. I was glad that we had learned these skills to employ. Still, I did not consider Brody to be a colicky baby. It is interesting, as expert as Jason and I had become in living and dealing with a colicky infant, we did not perceive our second child to be colicky. Maybe we were in denial. Maybe we felt like it was too soon to tell. Maybe we were fantasizing that it would go away. Maybe the fact that it felt different with Brody convinced us that it *was* different.

Brody never got as angry, upset, or worked up as Tyler did. He clearly was uncomfortable and cried because of it, but it was not all of the time nor was it nearly as intense or severe. In any case, it took other people to suggest that Brody could be colicky to make us really contemplate this possibility.

One of the people who proposed this possibility to us first was Tyler. There were many times that Tyler would come to Jason or me and say, "Brody cries a lot." Jason and I responded by saying, "Yes, that is one way babies talk to us." Tyler accepted this answer, but clearly became distraught over his cries. He knew something was bothering his baby brother. As I mentioned earlier, he often tried to console Brody. Interestingly, when this did not work, Tyler would join him. There were many car rides when Jason and I wanted to scream ourselves because our two boys were both screaming their heads off in the backseat.

My mother was the second person who alluded to the fact that Brody was not an easy baby. My mother and grandmother came out to visit when Brody was four weeks old. Jason was away on business and so they came to help me out with both of the kids. About halfway through the visit, my mother stated, "You have your hands full with these two boys." She proclaimed that Brody was a hard baby. She knew he was not nearly as hard as Tyler was, because she had experienced Tyler at the height of his colicky behavior. Nonetheless, she said Brody was "hard."

My cousin came to visit us for the weekend when my mother and grandmother were in town. I remember her telling me how crazy it was in our household. She was on the telephone with her own mother the next day asking her if it was that hard when she and her brother were Tyler and Brody's age.

When Brody turned five weeks old, I asked our child care provider what she thought of Brody's fussy behavior. She began helping me out with the kids when Brody was one week old. She had known Brody for one month when I approached her with this question. At first she seemed puzzled by my question and asked, "What do you mean?" She knew of our experiences with Tyler in the past. She also had a feel for both boys' temperaments and personalities in the present because she was there every weekday morning.

I explained to her that it was hard for me to know what normal baby behavior was since Tyler's newborn behavior was so extraordinary. In other words, Jason and I believed we had nothing to compare normal newborn behavior to. Brody was clearly easier. However, I wanted to get the perspective of someone who was not in my family on how easy or difficult Brody actually was. Due to the consistent time she spent with him and her expertise in the child care field, I thought she was the best to ask.

Her response surprised me. She said, "Brody is a really hard baby." In disbelief, I questioned, "Hard?" I then said, "You're kidding, right?" She said, "No, he is a colicky baby. He is fussy most of the time." I was stunned. I couldn't believe she used the word colic. It occurred to me for the first time that Brody's behavior was what most people would describe as colic. Our pediatrician later confirmed that Brody was colicky at his two-month appointment.

Having two kids under two is difficult. When one or both are colicky, it can feel impossible. Jason and I often joke about selling tickets for a weekend seminar at our house to expose certain populations to our insanity. Our target audience: teenagers who are having unprotected sex. We figured one weekend in our house with our two boys and our crazy lives would be a wonderful way to inspire teenagers to use contraceptives. We envisioned our flier to read: "Attention parents: Want to scare your child out of having unprotected sex? Have them spend a weekend with us. Free of charge. Baby-sitting duties will be required." Humor has always helped Jason and me cope with difficult times.

The good news is that like Tyler, Brody eventually outgrew his colic, which was much less severe and shorter lived. He was the "happiest baby on the block" by the age of ten and a half weeks. With Brody we did not even have to wait the one hundred days. Maybe this is because his discomfort was less or perhaps because his temperament from the beginning has been different from Tyler's. Brody is much better able to soothe himself. They are very different boys. Jason and I handled the stress of Brody's colicky cries differently because, in our minds, it was nothing compared to Tyler's.

As I said earlier, we thought we had it easy with Brody and never would have thought he was a colicky infant until this was confirmed by others. I suppose this conclusion speaks to all things being relative. At ten and a half weeks we could finally perceive and understand what it was like to have an easy baby. There is a sense of peacefulness when an infant is not screaming. We loved experiencing a newborn who smiled and cooed with the people around him. After Brody laughed for the first time (he was eleven weeks old), I remember saying to Jason, "Oh, I get it now. This is what everyone is talking about."

There is nothing more special and touching than having your newborn recognize you with a smile and a coo. It lifts your heart and mood in a way that only a parent can understand. Although I did not have this experience with Tyler when he was an infant, I am able to enjoy this experience with him now in his life and the feeling is exactly the same. Tyler can take my breath away with his smile and laughter. He is an unbelievably special little boy. I realize that our journey together created a bond between us that can never be broken and for that, I am extremely grateful.

As I mentioned earlier, I am a strong believer that things happen for a reason. Our family went through a very difficult time together and we came out on the other end stronger and more knowledgeable from the experience. The road back from this experience is what inspired me to write this book. I have met people since who have shared with me their own stories of the difficulties they faced with their newborn children. People *do* get through stressful and painful times.

There was one story that especially touched my heart, which I would like to share. After Tyler outgrew his colic, I decided to contact Pat to thank her for all of the help and support she provided to me and my family. She was glad that Tyler was doing better and asked if I would be willing to attend her support group the following week. She was interested in having me share my experiences with the new mothers in the group. I agreed to attend and was looking forward to it. I decided to bring Tyler with me that day. He was in a particularly good mood and was happy rolling around on the floor playing with his toys. It was hard to believe that only a few months earlier I was in that very same room with a screaming baby.

That day, approximately twenty women attended the support group meeting. After check-ins, Pat introduced me to the women and asked me to share my experiences with having a colicky infant. I introduced myself and Tyler to the group and then proceeded to tell the women what my experiences had been with Tyler only a few months earlier. The women found it hard to believe that the boy who lay in front of me chatting and smiling at everyone around him was the same boy I was describing in my story.

At the end of the meeting, I packed up Tyler and the diaper bag and started heading for the car. As I was leaving the room, a woman came up to me with tears streaming down her face. She asked if she could talk to me for a moment. She said that she could not believe the ordeal I had gone through with my son and quickly informed me that she was experiencing the same exact symptoms with her two-week-old. Pat had asked her to come to the support group meeting that day and she laughed. She said that it took every ounce of effort to leave her home that morning. She hadn't showered, eaten, or combed her hair. She didn't even have time to brush her teeth.

She went on to tell me how similar her son seemed to Tyler. She said that she was home alone with her infant while her husband worked long, hard hours. She did not have any family in the area and very few friends who lived close by. She stated that she felt isolated and alone. She also stated that she felt like a terrible parent and that she spent most of her days feeling like she was losing her mind because her son never stopped crying.

During our conversation, her son was sound asleep. However, as she became more emotional, he began to wake up. It was almost as if he sensed her disturbance. As he opened his eyes, he began to cry. His cries were soft at first, but then quickly escalated into full-fledged screams. I watched his mother as she tried to soothe him. Her face was strained. I could tell she was trying to hold back her tears and look lovingly at her child. She said, "Here he goes," and at that moment, her son began to shriek. He screamed so loud and hard that he had trouble catching his breath.

I knew these sounds all too well and it brought back many memories for me. My heart went out to this woman and to her baby. I knew that there was nothing I could say to her at that moment that would console her. However, I also knew that there were definitely things that I could do to lend her my support. I asked her if I could hold her baby. She looked up at me with a surprised look on her face. It was not a look of surprise due to her hesitation for her child's safety, but rather a look of surprise due to my interest and desire to hold her colicky child. I am sure she did not have many offers from other people to hold her son thus far. At least not while he was having what Jason and I often referred to as a "code red." Because I had lived through what she was currently suffering through with her infant, I knew how to respond.

I told her I wanted to illustrate some of the techniques that Jason and I often used with Tyler when he was in his worst colicky episodes. She was so pleased to gain some support, she handed her child over to me and watched me as I held him in my arms. First, I found a place to set him down and asked her for one of his blankets. I showed her how I swaddled Tyler and explained that the swaddle needed to be extremely tight or else her baby would find a way to get out of it. She told me swaddling never worked because her son was so strong that he could bust right out of the hold. We shared a smile as we joked about how strong colicky infants become due to their constant movement to find some comfort. I told her that Tyler held his head up sturdily by three weeks of age. He constantly kicked in his crib and on the changing table. He rolled over when he was two months old.

He sat up on his own at three and a half months. These were the things I told her she had to look forward to. I tried to give her some hope. I told her that what she was experiencing now would not last forever and that she would get through it.

I talked with her about the techniques we utilized to decrease Tyler's distress. I picked her screaming son up from the floor. He was clearly trying to break free from the swaddle he was in, and I turned him on his side, and began shushing in his ear. While shushing in his ear, I rocked him back and forth. Her son immediately melted in my arms. After a few minutes, I placed him in his car seat and slowly swung him back and forth as he gradually drifted back to sleep.

I was so involved with what I was doing, I was not paying attention to what was happening around me. Tyler was sitting in his car seat watching me and smiling from ear to ear. He had a toy in his hand and was talking to himself. Two other women who had not left the meeting yet came over to watch. I turned around to make eye contact with the baby's mother and found her in tears. Her facial expression was a mix of disbelief and gratitude. She could not speak. She did not have to. I knew exactly what she was thinking and feeling. I could feel her overwhelming emotion. I had been in that place many times before.

I set the car seat down on the floor beside her. She reached over and touched my arm. She whispered "thank you" in between her sobs. I could tell she was appreciative, but also embarrassed. I gently joked with her that after doing that ten times a day for over four months, you do become an expert. After talking to her for a few more moments about the techniques, I gave her my telephone number and told her to feel free to call me later that day if she needed any further support.

The group took place in the morning. I did not hear from the woman at all during the course of the day. I could not stop wondering how she and her baby were managing. At 9:00 p.m. that night the phone rang. I was in the middle of breast-feeding Tyler and could not pick up. After Tyler went to bed, I checked my messages. I was happy to hear the woman's voice on my answering machine.

She apologized for calling so late, but wanted to let me know how much she appreciated my help earlier that day. She stated that she was embarrassed about her outpouring of emotions but realized that I could most definitely understand what she was feeling. She informed me that after she left the group meeting she went directly to the bookstore to find some books on infant sleep and colic. She was surprised to find only two on the shelves: *The Happiest Baby on the Block* (Dr. Harvey Karp, Bantam) and *Secrets of the Baby Whisperer* (Tracy Hogg with Melinda Blau, Ballantine Books). She purchased both of them and then proceeded to go home. She did not think she would have any time to read the books, but surprisingly was able to read through the first several chapters of each. She stated, "My son slept solidly for four straight hours. I couldn't believe it."

She went on to say that when he had his next "code red," she utilized the techniques I showed her earlier that day and they worked well. Her son was currently asleep and had been sleeping for the past three hours. I could hear the relief in her voice. She ended her message to me by telling me I was her "angel." She stated that she believed that she was meant to be at the group meeting that she almost missed that morning and would be forever grateful that I was there on that same day to share my story with her. Hearing this woman's words was yet another confirmation that things do happen for a reason. Maybe sharing my experience will help individuals with difficult babies feel more supported and understood. It is not easy being a new parent. The adjustment to motherhood can be particularly complex.

Modern-day living is a balancing act. In most cases, both parents need to work to make ends meet. Parenting is a shared responsibility.

Being a working mother can be very difficult. In my case, I had responsibilities to fulfill at home as well as in my career. My family is a priority to me—that will never change. I feel privileged and blessed to have a career that is also a priority. My work is very important to me. Finding a way to balance all of these facets of my life has made me a stronger person. I am grateful for the opportunity to experience such richness in my life.

Experiencing first-time motherhood with a colicky infant was one of the hardest things that I have ever had to face. I have asked myself many times if I had it to do all over again, would I? The answer is yes. At the end of the storm there has always been a rainbow and that rainbow is Tyler. The months of hardship and heartache are gone. I will never forget them, but I don't dwell on them. I focus on the positive things that have taken place in my life since.

I often look at Tyler in awe. He is living proof that miracles happen. I love to watch him play baseball with his father in the backyard and see the excitement in his eyes every time he hits the ball "really far." I love to hear him say "watch me" before he tries something new. I love it when he says "let me do it" and then proceeds to accomplish tasks on his own. I love it when he looks at photographs in our home and tells me who is in each picture, along with a fond memory he has of that person.

I feel blessed every time he talks to his grandparents on the telephone and ends the conversation by telling them that he loves them and misses them. I love the fact that even though his uncles live far away, he never forgets special moments he has shared with them. I love it when he asks me how my day at work went. I love it when he wants me to tell him a story and then corrects me if I am telling it wrong. I love it when he learns a new word and uses it thirty times a day in the right context. What I love most of all is holding him in my arms and knowing that he is safe and healthy and secure. He has given me gifts that I could never give to myself. I am honored to experience the love shared by a mother and her child.

Index

D

E

emotional repercussions on parents, 20, 21, 22, 24, 37, 40, 43, 119, 125, 126, 151
anger, 35, 37, 41, 43, 116, 126, 135, 136, 158, 172
anxiety, v, 3, 18, 24, 43, 58, 59, 84, 127, 139, 140, 151, 172, 176, 190
distress, 1, 4, 8, 15, 18, 20, 24, 43, 46, 47, 49, 52, 54, 56, 58, 73, 77, 79, 83, 89, 95, 96, 97, 99, 102, 103, 106, 118, 126, 127, 133, 136, 139, 147, 151, 153, 156, 157, 161, 169, 179, 187, 191, 193, 204, 213
guilt, 133, 137, 141–143, 153, 154, 185
isolation, 4, 17, 24, 37, 38, 40, 59, 60, 128, 132, 137, 143–147, 152, 154, 170, 174, 177, 198
post-traumatic stress, 126
sleep deprivation, 5, 7, 137–141, 153, 155

F

Ferber, Dr. Richard, 35
Ferber technique, 35–36

G

GERD, 15, 16, 46, 50, 75–78, 80, 81, 100, 125
symptoms, 76, 100
treatment, 77, 78, 101
Babies Tum-Ease, 79
gripe water, 79
Mylicon drops, 79

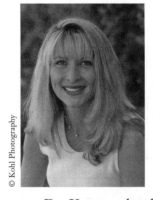

© Kohl Photography

Tonja H. Krautter, PsyD, LCSW, is a licensed clinical psychologist as well as a licensed clinical social worker. She has been practicing in the field of psychology for twelve years, developing an expertise in children and family issues. She has worked in hospital, residential, and day-treatment settings with extreme case matters, such as physical abuse, sexual assault, eating disorders, self-mutilation, suicide/homicide, substance abuse, and domestic violence.

Dr. Krautter has been in the role of clinical supervisor, program director, trainer, and workshop leader in a variety of settings. She is currently a private practitioner in Los Gatos, California, where she provides individual, family, and group therapy to her patients. Dr. Krautter is highly dedicated to the mental health field, serving persons in need and providing them with the highest standard of care. Dr. Krautter offers workshops and training seminars to a wide range of community agencies in the Bay Area. Seminar topics have included eating disorders, rape crisis and trauma, self-injurious behaviors, and therapy with special populations. She has published two journal articles in the *Journal of Family Therapy and Clinical Case Studies*. She is also currently writing a book for parents on self-injurious behavior that she hopes to bring to market in the near future.

Notes

Notes

Notes